D1174041

INFECTIOUS
WASTE
MANAGEMENT

HOW TO ORDER THIS BOOK

BY PHONE: 800-233-9936 or 717-291-5609, 8AM–5PM Eastern Time

BY FAX: 717-295-4538

BY MAIL: Order Department
Technomic Publishing Company, Inc.
851 New Holland Avenue, Box 3535
Lancaster, PA 17604, U.S.A.

BY CREDIT CARD: American Express, VISA, MasterCard

INFECTIOUS WASTE MANAGEMENT

Frank L. Cross, Jr., PE, DEE
President of Cross, Tessitore & Associates, PA, Orlando, FL

Howard E. Hesketh, Ph.D., PE, DEE
Professor of Engineering, Southern Illinois University, Carbondale, IL

P. Kay Rykowski, EIT
Project Engineer with Cross, Tessitore & Associates, PA, Orlando, FL

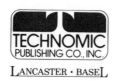

TECHNOMIC
PUBLISHING CO., INC.
LANCASTER · BASEL

Infectious Waste Management
a **TECHNOMIC**®publication

RA 567.7
.C76
1990

Published in the Western Hemisphere by
Technomic Publishing Company, Inc.
851 New Holland Avenue
Box 3535
Lancaster, Pennsylvania 17604 U.S.A.

Distributed in the Rest of the World by
Technomic Publishing AG

Copyright © 1990 by Technomic Publishing Company, Inc.
All rights reserved

No part of this publication may be reproduced, stored in a
retrieval system, or transmitted, in any form or by any means,
electronic, mechanical, photocopying, recording, or otherwise,
without the prior written permission of the publisher.

Printed in the United States of America
10 9 8 7 6 5 4 3 2 1

Main entry under title:
    Infectious Waste Management

A Technomic Publishing Company book
Bibliography: p.
Index: p. 149

Library of Congress Card No. 90-70714
ISBN No. 87762-751-7

Table of Contents

AUG 28 199

Preface

THE public is all too familiar with the unfortunate instances of environmental pollution caused by mismanagement of waste material, including infectious waste. The well publicized incidents where medical waste washed up on some of the nation's beaches have focused attention on proper management of infectious waste from hospitals, health care facilities, and other generators. This is not a new problem. Today, the problem is intensified because of liability issues, landfill laws, public concerns, and the tremendous increase in costs of handling transport and disposal of medical wastes. More comprehensive Joint Commission on Accreditation of Health-Care Organizations (JCAHO) requirements; environmental permitting, testing and reporting requirements of the Environmental Protection Agency (EPA) and state and local agencies; and new safety restrictions by the Occupational Safety and Health Administration (OSHA) have compounded confusion in establishing appropriate plans of action.

A considerable amount of information is available on the treatment and disposal procedures for hazardous wastes, but there is a deficiency of information on the subject of infectious waste. This book is written to help reduce this problem. Of the alternative techniques presently available for the destruction of medical wastes, incineration is usually the most acceptable because of disfiguration of the waste, volume reduction, pathogen destruction, and reduction in weight. All of these factors impact on the handling, transport, and disposal costs as well as the environmental impact and potential liability to the generator. The authors believe that this book will provide guidance to health care officials, their engineers, and their consultants concerning incineration, as well as other options for medical waste disposal.

The problem of infectious waste is described and defined in Chapter 1. With this material as background, Chapter 2 reviews a number of currently utilized practices plus several techniques being developed for treating and disposing of infectious wastes. Costs relative to these procedures are presented with other advantages and disadvantages. Recognizing that currently the most accepted treatment procedure is incineration, the remainder of the book (Chapters 3, 4 and 5) is devoted to presenting the technical and practical details and procedures relative to available and state-of-the-art systems.

Chapter 3 introduces details of incinerator waste feed, combustion requirements, incinerator principles, types of incinerators, refractory, regulations, and costs. Chapter 4 of this book has been devoted to the need for operator training as this is being required by many state regulatory agencies and is absolutely necessary to successfully operate and maintain the newer incinerators, energy recovery systems, air pollution control equipment, and monitoring instrumentation. Normal operation, start-up, shut-down, and upset procedures are presented in detail. Chapter 5 concludes by presenting information on energy recovery, regional (larger scale) uses, testing, and reporting. Material relative to economics is given as appropriate to incinerators (in Chapter 3) and regional systems (in Chapter 5).

The authors wish to thank Kyle Russell of the Missouri Department of Natural Resources for helping proofread the manuscript.

The Hospital Waste Problem

1.1 OVERVIEW

INFECTIOUS waste management is a problem that has been recognized for many years by environmental engineers and the health care industry. Only recently, however, has the subject come to the attention of the public and, consequently, local, state, and federal governments. Medical waste has evolved gradually over the years as medical practice has evolved. The waste stream is not much different today (early 1989) than it was five or ten years ago. Volume estimates are extremely variable (9–45 lbs/patient/day) [1]. The composition of the waste has also changed by the increase in plastic content (now 15–20 percent compared to 3–5 percent in community solid waste), and this higher plastic content makes incineration more difficult.

Waste handling consists primarily of manual collection systems with a variety of containers and hand-operated carts moving horizontally in corridors and vertically in elevators. The containers and transport systems used today remain relatively primitive in nature and have changed little from those used in the past. Treatment systems have also remained relatively traditional with limited modern innovation. Steam autoclaving (decontamination) remains a very effective way to render infectious waste safe for further handling and is the method of choice for laboratory cultures and other obviously infectious items. The alternative option is gaseous decontamination, primarily with ethylene oxide, but ethylene oxide itself is carcinogenic. Compacting for volume reduction has also generally been discouraged due to the potential for aerosolization and liquid leakage.

Other than the removal and transport of incineration effluent and biodegradation in landfills, disposal options are extremely limited. Grinding followed by liquid waste treatment in community sewage treatment facilities is currently practiced, but this option should be limited to the biodegradable portion of waste that is ultimately discharged to water systems in an innocuous, disinfected, and unrecognizable form. Nonbiodegradable plastics, glass, and metal can be burned in incinerators or buried in landfills. The following sections of this chapter discuss some of the procedures and problems associated with hospital waste disposal.

1.2 REGULATIONS FOR HANDLING, TRANSPORTING AND DISPOSING OF HOSPITAL WASTE

1.2.1 INFECTIOUS WASTE

Many local, state, and federal agencies are developing regulations concerning the management of infectious wastes. As of mid 1989, several states including New York, Pennsylvania, and Indiana already have programs in place. The movement to regulate the handling, transport, and disposal of infectious wastes actually started at the state level, with federal agencies slow to follow. The United States Environmental Protection Agency (USEPA) issued guidelines for infectious waste management in May, 1986, but has only recently directed a task force to develop infectious waste regulations [2]. The Occupational Safety and Health Association (OSHA) is expected to soon issue very comprehensive regulations on the handling of infectious wastes both within the health care facility and during transport and disposal.

The Medical Waste Tracking Act, passed by Congress into law on November 2, 1988, establishes record keeping and reporting requirements for generators, transporters, and facilities disposing of infectious waste. This will only, however, be a temporary program intended as a demonstration tracking system for medical waste. The legislation was essentially drafted as a result of public hysteria over the numerous occurrences of medical wastes washing up on beaches along the East Coast during the summer of 1988. The states of New York, New Jersey, Connecticut, and those bordering the Great Lakes were targeted for implementation of the regulations, although all fifty states were given the opportunity to "opt in" or "opt out" of the program. It is anticipated that this demonstration system will (1) prevent further washups of medical waste on the nation's beaches, (2) encourage safe, effective storage and disposal practices, and (3) provide information on how broader and more comprehensive regulations should be developed.

1.2.2 HAZARDOUS WASTE

While health care personnel must be concerned with the infectious waste they generate, they should also be aware that they may generate hazardous waste as well. Generation, storage, transport, treatment, and disposal of hazardous wastes are subject to the Resource Conservation and Recovery Act (RCRA) regulations. Those materials classified as hazardous wastes are clearly identified by these regulations. Typical hazardous wastes generated at a hospital or other health care facility are listed in Table 1.1.

The first group of wastes listed, antineoplastic drugs, is generated by most chemotherapy units. While there are many antineoplastic drugs used today, only those listed are classified as hazardous wastes. Some facilities, however, find it easier to handle all antineoplastic drug wastes as hazardous rather than trying to segregate them.

The second group of wastes listed, solvents, along with the third group, formaldehyde, are characteristic of pathological laboratory operations. Formaldehyde is classified as a hazardous waste only if it is discarded in its unused form. For example, if a portion of a container of the substance was used and the remainder discarded, the remaining portion would be considered a hazardous waste. However, if a quantity of formaldehyde was used to preserve a lab specimen or tissue and then discarded, it would not be considered hazardous. The RCRA regulations provide separate listings of wastes in their used and unused forms, and many substances are included in both. Formaldehyde is listed only as an unused material. In addition to specific listings of wastes in various forms as hazardous, the regulations define five characteristics of hazardous wastes. Any waste that is not listed specifically but still meets any of these five characteristics is also considered hazardous. Used formaldehyde discarded in its pure form would meet the characteristic of ignitability, and therefore would be classified as hazardous. However, formaldehyde used in most health care facilities is actually a solution containing 30 to 50 percent water, which lowers the flash point and thus limits its ignitability.

TABLE 1.1 Typical Hazardous Waste Generated at Medical/Health Care Facilities.

---

1. **ANTINEOPLASTIC DRUGS**
   - Chlorambucil
   - Cyclophosphamide (Cytoxin)
   - Daunomycin
   - Mitomycin C
   - Streptozotocin (Zanosar)
   - Melphalan
   - Uracil Mustard

2. **SOLVENTS**
   - Xylene
   - Toluene

3. **FORMALDEHYDE (UNUSED)**

TABLE 1.2 Categories of Hazardous Waste Generators.

Very Small Quantity (or conditionally exempt small quantity) Generators	Small Quantity Generators	Generators
Generate no more than 100 kg (about 220 lbs or 25 gals) of hazardous waste in any calendar month.	Generate more than 100 and less than 1000 kg of hazardous waste in any calendar month.	Generate 1000 kg (about 2200 lbs or 300 gallons) or more of hazardous waste any any calendar month.
Never accumulate more than 1000 kg of hazardous waste on facility property.		

Under RCRA regulations, generators of hazardous waste are subject to different standards according to the quantity of waste generated per month. Table 1.2 provides a guide to the classification by size category of hazardous waste generators, while Table 1.3 provides an overview of RCRA requirements for small quantity generators. Sample "Notification of Hazardous Waste Activity" and "Uniform Hazardous Waste Manifest" forms are included in Tables 1.4 and 1.5 respectively.

1.3 CHARACTERIZATION OF HOSPITAL WASTE

Wastes generated at health care facilities are indeed varied both in composition and in quantity. Hospitals offer a wide range of services and en-

TABLE 1.3 Overview of Small Quantity Generator Requirements.

1. Obtain a USEPA Identification Number by submitting "Notification of Hazardous Waste Activity" Form
2. Comply with hazardous waste transportation requirements
   a. U.S. Department of Transportation (DOT) packaging, labeling, marking, and placarding requirements
      —Packaging requirements in 49 CFR Parts 173, 178, & 179
      —Labeling and marking requirements in 49 CFR Part 172 (for both on-site storage and transporting wastes off-site)
      —Placarding requirements of 49 CFR Part 172, subpart F
      Publications containing these DOT regulations may be obtained from: The Superintendent of Documents, U.S. Government Printing Office, Washington, D.C., 20402
   b. Hazardous waste must be transported by a licensed hazardous waste transporter.
3. Annually report on Hazardous Waste activity

TABLE 1.4 Sample "Notification of Hazardous Waste Activity" Form.

For Official Use Only

													Comments														
C																											
C																											

	Installation's EPA ID Number										T/A	C	Approved	Date Received (yr. mo. day)		
C												1				
F																

I. Name of Installation

G	E	N	E	R	A	L		M	E	T	A	L		P	R	O	C	E	S	S	I	N	G		C	O	

II. Installation Mailing Address

Street or P.O. Box
C 3	5	0	1		M	A	I	N		S	T														

	City or Town															State		ZIP Code		
C 4	S	M	A	L	L	T	O	W	N							V	A	2 3 0 0 0		

III. Location of Installation

Street or Route Number
C 5	5	0	1		M	A	I	N		S	T														

	City or Town															State		ZIP Code		
C 6	S	M	A	L	L	T	O	W	N							V	A	2 3 0 0 0		

IV. Installation Contact

Name and Title (last, first, and job title)
																Phone Number (area code and number)		
C 2	J	O	N	E	S		W	I	L	L	I	A	M		M	G R	8 0 4	5 5 5 0 5 0 9

V. Ownership

A. Name of Installation's Legal Owner
														B. Type of Ownership (enter code)
C R	D	O	E		J	O	S	E	P	H	I	N	E	P

VI. Type of Regulated Waste Activity *(Mark 'X' in the appropriate boxes. Refer to instructions.)*

A. Hazardous Waste Activity	B. Used Oil Fuel Activities
☒ 1a. Generator ☒ 1b. Less than 1,000 kg/mo.	☐ 6. Off-Specification Used Oil Fuel
☐ 2. Transporter	*(enter 'X' and mark appropriate boxes below)*
☐ 3. Treater/Storer/Disposer	☐ a. Generator Marketing to Burner
☐ 4. Underground Injection	☐ b. Other Marketer
☐ 5. Market or Burn Hazardous Waste Fuel	☐ c. Burner
(enter 'X' and mark appropriate boxes below)	☐ 7. Specification Used Oil Fuel Marketer (or On site Burner)
☐ a. Generator Marketing to Burner	Who First Claims the Oil Meets the Specification
☐ b. Other Marketer	
☐ c. Burner	

VII. Waste Fuel Burning: Type of Combustion Device *(enter 'X' in all appropriate boxes to indicate type of combustion device(s) in which hazardous waste fuel or off-specification used oil fuel is burned. See instructions for definitions of combustion devices.)*

☐ A. Utility Boiler   ☐ B. Industrial Boiler   ☐ C. Industrial Furnace

VIII. Mode of Transportation *(transporters only — enter 'X' in the appropriate box(es)*

☐ A. Air   ☐ B. Rail   ☐ C. Highway   ☐ D. Water   ☐ E. Other *(specify)*

IX. First or Subsequent Notification

Mark 'X' in the appropriate box to indicate whether this is your installation's first notification of hazardous waste activity or a subsequent notification. If this is not your first notification, enter your installation's EPA ID Number in the space provided below.

☒ A. First Notification   ☐ B. Subsequent Notification *(complete item C)*

C. Installation's EPA ID Number											

EPA Form 8700-12 (Rev. 11-85) Previous edition is obsolete.

(continued)

5

TABLE 1.4 (Continued).

X. Description of Hazardous Wastes *(continued from front)*

A. Hazardous Wastes from Nonspecific Sources. Enter the four-digit number from 40 *CFR* Part 261.31 for each listed hazardous waste from nonspecific sources your installation handles. Use additional sheets if necessary.

1	2	3	4	5	6
F 0 0 8	F 0 1 1				
7	8	9	10	11	12

B. Hazardous Wastes from Specific Sources. Enter the four-digit number from 40 *CFR* Part 261.32 for each listed hazardous waste from specific sources your installation handles. Use additional sheets if necessary.

13	14	15	16	17	18
K 0 6 9					
19	20	21	22	23	24
25	26	27	28	29	30

C. Commercial Chemical Product Hazardous Wastes. Enter the four-digit number from 40 *CFR* Part 261.33 for each chemical substance your installation handles which may be a hazardous waste. Use additional sheets if necessary.

31	32	33	34	35	36
37	38	39	40	41	42
43	44	45	46	47	48

D. Listed Infectious Wastes. Enter the four-digit number from 40 *CFR* Part 261.34 for each hazardous waste from hospitals, veterinary hospitals, or medical and research laboratories your installation handles. Use additional sheets if necessary.

49	50	51	52	53	54

E. Characteristics of Nonlisted Hazardous Wastes. Mark 'X' in the boxes corresponding to the characteristics of nonlisted hazardous wastes your installation handles. *(See 40 CFR Parts 261.21 — 261.24)*

☐ 1. Ignitable (D001)   ☐ 2. Corrosive (D002)   ☐ 3. Reactive (D003)   ☐ 4. Toxic (D000)

XI. Certification

I certify under penalty of law that I have personally examined and am familiar with the information submitted in this and all attached documents, and that based on my inquiry of those individuals immediately responsible for obtaining the information, I believe that the submitted information is true, accurate, and complete. I am aware that there are significant penalties for submitting false information, including the possibility of fine and imprisonment.

Signature	Name and Official Title *(type or print)*	Date Signed
Josephine Doe	JOSEPHINE DOE OWNER	6/1/86

EPA Form 8700-12 (Rev. 11-85) Reverse

6

TABLE 1.5 Sample "Uniform Hazardous Waste Manifest" Form.

Please print or type   (Form designed for use on elite (12-pitch) typewriter)   Form Approved OMB No 2000-0404 Expires 7-31-86

UNIFORM HAZARDOUS WASTE MANIFEST	1 Generator's US EPA ID No V A D 0 0 1 2 3 4 5 6 7	Manifest Document No 0 0 0 0 7	2 Page 1 of	Information in the shaded areas is not required by Federal law.

			A. State Manifest Document Number

3 Generator's Name and Mailing Address
GENERAL METAL PROCESSING CO.
501 MAIN ST.
SMALLTOWN, VA 23000

B State Generator's ID

4 Generator's Phone (804) 555-0509

5 Transporter 1 Company Name SAFETY HAULER	6 US EPA ID Number V A D 0 0 8 9 1 2 3 4 5	C. State Transporter's ID

D. Transporter's Phone

7 Transporter 2 Company Name	8 US EPA ID Number	E State Transporter's ID

F. Transporter's Phone

9 Designated Facility Name and Site Address DISPOS-ALL, INC 1800 NORTH AVE FRIENDLY TOWN, VA 23000	10 US EPA ID Number V A D 0 0 0 6 7 8 9 1 2 3	G State Facility's ID

H. Facility's Phone

11 US DOT Description (Including Proper Shipping Name, Hazard Class, and ID Number)	12 Containers		13 Total Quantity	14 Unit Wt/Vol	I. Waste No
	No	Type			
a. HAZARDOUS WASTE, LIQUID OR SOLID, NOS ORM-E, NA9189	0 0 2	DM	0 0 1 1 0	GAL	
b. WASTE CYANIDE SOLUTION, NOS UN1935	0 0 1	DM	0 0 0 5 5	GAL	
c. WASTE FLAMMABLE LIQUID, NOS UN1993	0 0 1	DM	0 0 0 5 5	GAL	
d.					

J. Additional Descriptions for Materials Listed Above

K. Handling Codes for Wastes Listed Above

15 Special Handling Instructions and Additional Information

16 GENERATOR'S CERTIFICATION: I hereby declare that the contents of this consignment are fully and accurately described above by proper shipping name and are classified, packed, marked, and labeled, and are in all respects in proper condition for transport by highway according to applicable international and national government regulations

Unless I am a small quantity generator who has been exempted by statute or regulation from the duty to make a waste minimization certification under Section 3002(b) of RCRA, I also certify that I have a program in place to reduce the volume and toxicity of waste generated to the degree I have determined to be economically practicable and I have selected the method of treatment, storage, or disposal currently available to me which minimizes the present and future threat to human health and the environment

Printed/Typed Name JOSEPHINE K. DOE	Signature Josephine K. Doe	Month Day Year 10 8 30 86

17 Transporter 1 Acknowledgement of Receipt of Materials		
Printed/Typed Name	Signature	Month Day Year

18 Transporter 2 Acknowledgement of Receipt of Materials		
Printed/Typed Name	Signature	Month Day Year

19 Discrepancy Indication Space

20 Facility Owner or Operator Certification of receipt of hazardous materials covered by this manifest except as noted in Item 19		
Printed/Typed Name	Signature	Month Day Year

EPA Form 8700-22 (Rev. 4-85) Previous edition is obsolete

Information in the shaded areas is not required by Federal law, but this or other additional information may be required by your state.

TABLE 1.6 **Infectious Wastes.**

- Cultures and stocks of infectious agents and associated pathologicals
- Pathological wastes of human origin
- Pathological wastes of animal origin that have been exposed to infectious agents
- Blood and blood products
- Blood soaked gauze, bandages, sponges and other materials
- Containers used to hold blood
- Sharps, including syringes, scalpel blades, needles with attached tubing, and broken or unbroken glassware that has contacted infectious agents
- Bedding materials of animals that have been exposed to infectious agents
- Isolation wastes or discarded materials used in the care of human beings or animals who are isolated to protect others from certain highly communicable diseases

compass a variety of activities, each of which generates a different characteristic waste. Other health care or health-related facilities may be more one-dimensional in the services offered and therefore generate a more limited waste stream.

It is important to know what types and quantities of waste are generated at a facility for several reasons. Some state and local governments have implemented waste generation reporting requirements for hospitals. Proper sizing of an on-site treatment system requires an accurate characterization of the waste generated. Some contracts for transportation and off-site disposal of waste are based on the quantity generated as well.

For these requirements, the most accurate method of gathering data is to conduct a facility waste audit. This can be accomplished by in-house personnel or by an environmental engineering consulting firm specializing in infectious and solid waste management. The following sections, however, provide general information including the types, composition, and physical and chemical characteristics of wastes generated at health care facilities.

1.3.1 TYPES OF HOSPITAL WASTES

The types of wastes generated at a health care facility can be classified into three general categories: (1) infectious or biohazardous waste, (2) noninfectious solid waste, and (3) hazardous waste.

Low Level Radioactive wastes are a fourth waste stream that is handled and disposed of in a dependable manner separate from the other wastes.

Recently, infectious or biohazardous waste has been the focus of much concern. The term infectious waste is, however, somewhat nebulous in that there is no universally known definition of the category. Every local, state, and federal program that regulates infectious waste develops its own definition. Table 1.6 provides a list of items normally labeled as infectious when they appear in the waste stream. The U.S. Environmental Protection

Agency first promulgated enforceable definitions of infectious waste in March 1989 in the Medical Waste Tracking Act of 1988. This act listed the following ten categories of regulated medical waste:

(1) Cultures and stocks of infectious agents

(2) Pathological wastes (tissues, organs, body parts)

(3) Blood and other body fluids

(4) Contaminated sharps

(5) Animal body parts

(6) Surgery wastes

(7) Laboratory wastes

(8) Dialysis wastes

(9) Contaminated medical equipment and biological waste

(10) Materials contaminated by contact with bodily fluids

These regulations only define which items need to be tracked and do not specify what waste types are actually infectious and should be treated.

In 1978, EPA guidelines suggested that 20–25 percent of hospital waste should be considered as infectious. In contrast, the Centers for Disease Control (CDC) consider only 3–5 percent of hospital waste as infectious [6]. Subtitle C of the RCRA defines hazardous waste so as to include solid waste with infectious characteristics.

Infectious waste regulation has increased dramatically from 1988 to 1990. Greater volumes of material considered as infectious waste are being generated. Tougher incinerator air emission standards and ash and landfill regulations make it important to recognize the problem and to solve it effectively.

Noninfectious solid waste generated at health care facilities include many items found in municipal solid waste. Many hospitals have accounting, record keeping, purchasing, engineering, and administrative services that produce wastes characteristic of typical office activities. Cafeteria or food service operations generate relatively large quantities of food scraps and food packaging materials. Depending on the regulations considered, most wastes generated from patient care activities may be considered

TABLE 1.7 **Noninfectious Solid Wastes.**

- Cardboard
- Paper documents, boxed or loose
- Discarded linens
- Disposable food packaging and containers
- Food scraps
- Foam mattresses, or "egg crates"

noninfectious as long as no exposure to infectious agents occurred. Table 1.7 provides a list of items typically included in noninfectious solid waste generated at a health care facility.

A third type of waste generated at many health care facilities is hazardous waste. Generation of significant quantities of hazardous waste is subject to record keeping and reporting requirements set forth by the Resource Conservation and Recovery Act regulations (see section 1.2). Refer to Table 1.1 for a list of typical hazardous wastes generated at a health care facility.

1.3.2 COMPOSITION OF HOSPITAL WASTES

The waste stream generated at health care facilities is extremely heterogeneous in composition; however, it can be generally described as a mixture of paper and cardboard, plastic, pathological waste, food waste, glass, and metal. Factors affecting the amount of these elements present in the waste stream include the extent of laboratory and/or research activities, use of disposables, and the rate of surgeries scheduled.

Table 1.8 shows the approximate composition of various wastes generated at health care facilities. This distribution changes with time, and the current trend is toward the use of more plastics.

1.3.3 PHYSICAL/CHEMICAL CHARACTERISTICS

In order to optimize waste management practices at a health care facility, it is often necessary to consider the physical and chemical characteris-

TABLE 1.8 Waste Composition.

Types of Operation	% Paper	% Plastic	% Pathological	% Foodwaste	% Glass	% Metal	% Other
• Administrative/Clerical	100	—	—	—	—	—	—
• Cafeteria	20	20	—	30	—	—	—
• Surgery	60	30	10	—	—	—	—
• Emergency Room	60	35	5	—	—	—	—
• Intensive Care	60	35	5	—	—	—	—
• Renal Dialysis	10	85	5	—	—	—	—
• Laboratory	35	30	25	—	10	—	—
• Nursery	45	35	—	5	15	—	—
• Pharmacy	50	30	—	—	20	—	—
• General Patient Care	60	35	—	5	—	—	—
• Research	40	—	30	—	—	—	20*
• Sharps	—	90	—	—	—	10	—

*Animal Bedding

tics of the waste stream. Table 1.9 lists the characteristics of several waste types that are included in the waste stream generated at health care facilities. Table 1.10 includes an analysis of plastics found in the waste stream along with examples of the two composite mixtures.

1.4 WASTE HANDLING

The subject of infectious waste management is often focused on issues relating to disposal; however, in developing proper management practices, waste handling procedures used throughout the health care facility should be considered as well.

Waste handling practices should be designed to meet two primary objectives: (1) to achieve a free flowing path for the movement of waste from generation to disposal and (2) to minimize risk to personnel.

The first objective is relatively fundamental. It may be accomplished simply by identifying points of generation and providing adequate storage areas for accumulation of wastes until on-site treatment and/or off-site transportation occurs. For some large facilities, it may be helpful to devise a waste flow chart to develop an effective waste management plan.

As indicated in section 1.2, the Occupational Safety and Health Administration is expected to issue very comprehensive regulations on handling of infectious wastes both within the health care facility and during transportation and disposal.

Currently, most waste handlers wear latex gloves as personal protective equipment, and while this practice provides no protection against needle sticks, it does provide a barrier to prevent direct contact with infectious agents. Most state regualtions require packaging of infectious waste in red or orange bags, with the labels "Infectious" or "Biohazardous" clearly affixed. Carts are often used, very effectively, for transporting wastes within the facility. Sharps should be disposed of in rigid plastic containers with lids to protect handlers from sticks. Overfilling is a common problem with sharps containers that may cause needles to protrude from openings and lids to become detached. Care should be taken to ensure the proper use of any waste container. Proper handling of used sharps is perhaps the most important issue in reducing risk to health care workers and has been the focus of increased public attention, due largely to the general hysteria accompanying the rise of Acquired Immune Deficiency Syndrome (AIDS) as a public health problem during the 1980s. As long as sufficient efforts are made at the point of generation to segregate sharps from the general medical waste stream and then to safely package and transfer them to a disposal site, risks should be minimized.

A third concern, which may be secondary in nature in establishing waste handling practices, is aesthetics. Waste generated at health care facilities

TABLE 1.9 **Waste Types** [3].

Classification of Wastes			Principal Components	Approximate Composition (% by Weight)	Moisture Content (% by Weight)	Incombustible Solids (% by Weight)	Heating Value (BTU Value/Lb of Refuse as Fired)
Type	Description						
Class 0	Trash		Highly combustible waste. Paper, wood, cardboard cartons and up to 10% treated papers, plastic or rubber scraps: commercial and industrial sources.	Trash 100	10	5	8500
Class 1	Rubbish		Combustible waste, paper, cartons, rags, wood scraps, combustible floor sweepings: domestic, commercial and industrial sources.	Garbage 20	25	10	6500
Class 2	Refuse		Rubbish and garbage: residential sources	Rubbish 50 Garbage 50	50	7	4800
Class 3	Garbage		Animal and vegetable wastes; restaurants, hotels, markets, institutional, commercial, and club sources	Garbage 65 Rubbish 35	70	5	2500
Class 4	Animal solids and organics		Carcasses, organs, solid organic wastes: hospital, laboratory, abattoirs, animal pounds and similar sources	Animal and human tissue 100	85	5	1000

TABLE 1.10 Plastics Analysis [4,5].

	Paper	Poly-Ethylene (PE)	Poly-Styrene (PS)	Poly-Urethane (PU)	Polyvinyl Chloride (PVC)
Carbon	41.68	84.38	86.74	63.14	45.04
Hydrogen	5.87	14.14	8.42	6.25	5.60
Oxygen	35.76	0.00	3.96	17.61	1.56
Nitrogen	0.29	0.06	0.21	5.98	0.08
Sulfur	0.20	0.03	0.02	0.02	0.14
Chlorine	0.00	0.00	0.00	2.42	45.32
Moisture	10.20	0.20	0.20	0.20	0.20
Ash	6.00	1.19	0.45	4.38	2.06
Total	100.00	100.00	100.00	100.00	100.00
HHV[a], MEAS.	7572	19687	16419	11203	9754
HHV, CALC.	7557	20401	17286	11566	9693

Composite Hospital Waste Examples with Different Moisture and Ash (Combustables in each are 75% paper; 25% plastic, e.g., 16.21% PE, 1.9% PS, 1.1% PU, 5.79% PVC)

Carbon	49.78		42.80
Hydrogen	7.25		6.22
Oxygen	27.18		23.32
Nitrogen	0.30		0.26
Sulfur	0.16		0.14
Chlorine	2.65		2.27
Moisture	7.70		10.00
Ash	4.87		15.00
Total	~100.00		~100.00

Composite Average HHV 9991 Btu/lb   Composite Average HHV 8500 Btu/lb

[a]HHV—High Heating Value, Btu/lb

may be offensive to both sight and smell. Offenses may be avoided, however, through proper packaging and timely disposal schedules. A variety of opaque, rigid plastic containers are available for handling pathological wastes and/or large volumes of blood and blood products. Red bags traditionally used for infectious wastes should conceal the appearance of most items they may contain. Separate housing structures dedicated solely to on-site storage may be used for temporary housing of wastes before either on-site disposal or off-site transportation occurs. In some cases, refrigerated storage may be required if wastes must be stored for an extended period of time.

Some health care facilities may be required to develop a formal waste management plan in which waste handling procedures for all waste types are outlined specifically. Even if not required, this plan may be a positive step in developing waste handling procedures as required by the transportation, treatment, and disposal methods used. Proper waste handling procedures can be extremely effective in calming fears resulting from the increasing public scrutiny of the medical waste problem.

1.5 SUMMARY

When the subject of infectious waste is raised, inevitably the question, "What is infectious waste?" is asked. It is an important question because its answer impacts all aspects of infectious waste management, including transportation, storage, treatment, and disposal. It is also a question that has become the focus of much regulatory concern.

This chapter provides a summary of currently available information on the characteristics of various types of waste generated at health care facilities. While defining truly "infectious" waste will require a consensus from the scientific community, the information provided here may be used to attain a more educated perspective on medical waste in general.

REFERENCES

1 U.S. Congress, Office of Technology Assessment. *Issues in Medical Waste Management—Background Paper.* OTA-BP-O-49. Washington, D.C.:U.S. Government Printing Office (October 1988).

2 U.S. Environmental Protection Agency, Office of Solid Waste and Emergency Response. *EPA Guide for Infectious Waste Management.* EPA/530-SW-86-014. Springfield, VA:National Technical Information Service (May 1986).

3 Cross, F. L. and H. E. Hesketh. *Controlled Air Incineration.* Lancaster, PA:Technomic Publishing Co. (1985).

4 Perry, J. H., ed. *Chemical Engineers Handbook*, 6th edition. New York:McGraw-Hill (1984).

5 Radian Corporation. *Hospital Waste Combustion Study—Data Gathering Phase.* EPA No. 68-02-4330 (October 1987).

6 Hoffman, S. L. and N. J. Cabral. "Solving the Problems of Infectious Waste Disposal," *Solid Waste and Power*, 3(3):24–30 (June 1989).

Methods of Treatment and Disposal

2.1 COMPARISON OF METHODS

THE purpose of treatment is to change the biological character of the waste to eliminate, or at least to significantly reduce, its potential for causing damage. The two most common techniques used to treat infectious wastes are incineration and steam sterilization. Other currently available techniques include compaction, hydropulping, and microwaving. Other emerging and existing technologies include sterilization/grinding, direct irradiation, and distillation. Table 2.1 compares some of these procedures. For various treatment processes, Table 2.2 shows how the initial weight of 500 lb of material is reduced and Table 2.3 shows how the initial volume of 100 yd³ is reduced following treatment [1].

Capital and operating costs for some of these technologies are given in Table 2.4; however, keep in mind that the data from the preceding tables show that all processes do not yield the same final results. Advantages and disadvantages are summarized for these technologies in Table 2.5.

Table 2.6 is a comparison between the two most popular techniques, steam sterilization/compaction and incineration, and lists potential environmental impacts for the two. With sterilization, the key to minimizing environmental impact is proper operation of the system. Sharps and other contaminated wastes must be carefully handled to assure proper feed to the system. Densely packed wastes must be redistributed to allow sufficient exposure to steam. A rigid testing program utilizing spore strips routinely placed throughout the waste stream must be enacted. If these procedures are not followed, sterilization of infectious wastes may not be effective, and this negligence could result in a release of infectious agents to the environment.

Proper operating conditions are also important in preventing adverse environmental effects of incineration. Sufficient temperatures and combustion air levels must be maintained in the combustion chambers to ensure

TABLE 2.1 Alternative Solutions for Waste Treatment Techniques.

Methods	Technique	Waste Types Suitable for Treatment				
		Pathological	Administrative (Type 0)	Hazardous (1)	Infectious	Food Service (Type 3)
Radiation	Electromagnetic (Microwave)				■	
	Direct Irradiation (Cobalt-60)				■	
Oxidation	Incineration	■	■	■	■	■
	Hydropulping	■			■	
Sterilization	Steam Injection				■	
	Ethylene Chloride (2)				■	
Pretreatment	Compaction				■	
Combination	Sterilization/ Compaction				■	
	Sterilization/Grinding				■	

Notes: (1) Xylene, Toluene, Benzene, Formaldehyde, Chemotherapy, etc. (2) No longer used due to very restrictive standards for operation.

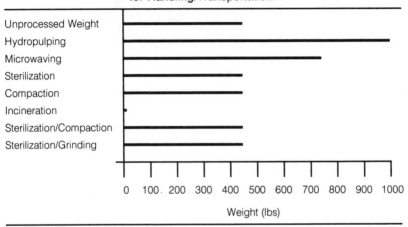

TABLE 2.2 How Systems Alter the Weight of Waste
for Handling/Transportation.

Weight (lbs)

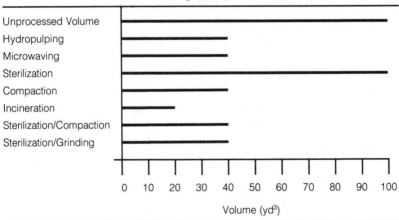

TABLE 2.3 How Systems Alter the Volume of Waste
for Handling/Transportation.

Volume (yd³)

17

TABLE 2.4 Cost Comparison of Medical Waste Treatment Technologies.

	Operation & Maintenance ($/lb/h)	Capital Equipment ($/lb/h)
Incineration	0.04	500.00[1]
Hydropulping	0.06	200.00
Microwaving	0.15	750.00
Sterilization	0.07	300.00
Sterilization/Compaction	0.08	400.00
Sterilization/Grinding	0.08	500.00

EXAMPLE:

500 lb/h Incinerator

—Capital Cost
500 lb/h × $500/lb/h = $250,000

—Operating Cost
Assume 12 h operating day
500 lb/h × $0.04/lb/h × 12 h/day × 365 days/y = $8,760/y

[1]Controlled-Air Incinerator

TABLE 2.5 Advantages and Disadvantages of
Waste Handling/Disposal Techniques.

System	Advantages	Disadvantages
Incineration	• maximum volume weight reduction	• noncombustibles not reduced in volume (ash, metal, etc.)
	• sterile residue when operated properly	• complex operation considering environmental factors
	• moderate amount of space required	• requires trained operator
	• air emissions can be controlled	• non-combustibles and ash may pose disposal problem
		• auxiliary fuel required
Hydropulping	• reduction in volume	• adds substantial weight to product for disposal
	• should provide good disinfection	• difficult for biomonitoring
	• substantially changes appearance of waste	• chlorine solution discharged to POTW[1] may not be acceptable
Sterilization (Autoclaving)	• low cost (capital & operating)	• may have increased waste handling

TABLE 2.5 (Continued).

System	Advantages	Disadvantages
	• low maintenance	• need thorough testing program (spore strip testing) • no volume reduction • no change in appearance of waste
Direct Irradiation	• positive disinfection, very reliable for providing good disinfection	• not demonstrated for infectious waste treatment • permitting expensive and special licenses required • high capital cost • extensive monitoring required • no volume reduction
Compaction	• reduces volume of waste • relatively inexpensive	• does not reduce weight • no disinfection • may not render sharps unusable • may cause leakage problem • may cause difficulty in incineration or other treatment
Microwaving	• reduces volume of waste (because of grinding) • moderate cost	• may result in fugitive emissions of volatile organic compounds (VOC) • requires strict monitoring program • biomonitoring difficult
Sterilization/ Compaction	• positive disinfection • good volume reduction • low cost • results in change in appearance of waste	• difficult to perform biomonitoring • no weight reduction
Sterilization/ Grinding	• low cost • good volume reduction • substantially changes appearance of waste • positive disinfection • not difficult to perform biomonitoring	• moderate maintenance required

[1]Publicly owned treatment works (municipal wastewater treatment plant)

TABLE 2.6 Potential Environmental Risks/Concerns.

Steam Sterilization/Compaction	Incineration
—No destruction of organics (possible release to air through vent)	—Potential release of particulates, acid gases to air (these are regulated)
—No regulation of operating methods	—Ash may contain heavy metals (depending on waste stream)
—No disfigurement of waste	
—Any laxity in testing program could result in release of infectious waste	
—Sharps may remain in usable condition	

destruction of organics. However, as long as incinerators are equipped with auxiliary burners, the temperature can be automatically controlled.

Aesthetics is an important issue in the handling and treatment of waste and is especially true for medical facilities because they are often located in conspicuous places in the local community. Infectious wastes are generally displeasing to both site and smell. Even though both steam sterilization/compaction and incineration are effective in treating infectious wastes, they evoke quite different aesthetic concerns.

Steam sterilization/compaction does not substantially change the appearance of the infectious waste. Blood, blood products, body tissues and fluids remain recognizable, and the sight of these waste types in a public landfill disturbs many people. Hypodermic needles and other sharps are physically unchanged by the process and may also be considered objectionable. The steam sterilization process itself is characterized by a very acrid smell, which may be offensive if present near hospital operations. In addition, if treated waste is compacted, it will almost always sit in a compactor on or near hospital grounds for some length of time while waiting to be landfilled, and this delay could result in the release of foul odors.

Incineration is the one treatment technique that actually destroys waste materials. The resulting ash residue is generally indistinguishable from that of an ordinary fireplace. However, insufficient operating conditions and inferior equipment may result in poor "burnout" of the ash, that is, some subjects may not be burned completely and may be at least partially recognizable when discharged to the ash pit. This condition most often occurs when an incinerator is loaded beyond capacity. Poor burnout is a symptom of a problem and should never be allowed to continue for an extended period of time.

The more common aesthetic concern with incineration involves the exhaust gas vented to the atmosphere. When certain wastes are burned, such as chlorinated plastics, the exhaust gas may take on an unpleasant odor due to the formation of acidic compounds during combustion. Exhaust gases may also appear black in color and/or in varying degrees of opacity. These problems can be easily corrected by adding a control device to the system, such as a fabric filter or lime scrubber. It should be noted that careful, attentive operators can do much to improve the aesthetic qualities of any waste treatment process.

Economics, aesthetics, and environmental issues are certainly important in choosing an infectious waste treatment system; however, they become meaningless if the technology itself is not effective. For both steam sterilization and incineration, careful operation is the key to system effectiveness. This point is important, because the consequences of system failure could be serious. The purpose of treating infectious waste is to eliminate the disease-causing potential of infectious agents contained in the waste. Failure to accomplish this could result in the release of pathogens to the environment and to individuals handling the waste.

2.2 INCINERATION

Incineration utilizes combustion to reduce waste materials to noncombustible residue or ash and exhaust gases. This process actually serves as both treatment and disposal of wastes. Infectious agents are killed by the excessive temperatures reached in the incinerator, exhaust gases are vented to the atmosphere, and only the ash must be landfilled.

Incineration is a suitable technology for the treatment of all types of infectious wastes. Incineration utilizes combustion to effect treatment. Operating conditions greatly affect system performance; however, unlike steam sterilization, an incinerator system may be monitored visually by observing ash quality and air emissions. A decrease in temperature, obstruction of the air flow to waste, or improper mixing of the waste may result in poor burnout of the ash and/or excessive air emissions. Keys to maintaining proper system performance include the following:

(1) Incineration design including a secondary burning chamber
(2) Use of auxiliary fuel-fired burners to maintain a temperature of at least 1,600°F in the primary and 1,800–2,000°F in the secondary chamber
(3) Minimum exhaust gas residence time of 1–2 seconds in the secondary chamber
(4) Proper residence time to obtain complete burnout
(5) Regulated combustion air

These measures would preclude problems typically associated with hard-to-burn wastes such as pathological waste, food waste, and plastic-filled sharps containers. Volume reduction achieved by a properly run incinerator is approximately 95 percent. This technology is highly effective at treating infectious wastes.

Today and perhaps for the short term (i.e., the next five to ten years), incineration will remain the preferred method for the treatment of medical wastes. The advantages of this technology include the following:

- suitable for all types of medical wastes (including pathological, laboratory, and hazardous waste types)
- provides substantial reduction in volume and weight
- produces a sterile ash/noncombustible residue for disposal

Air emissions can be substantially reduced with the addition of air pollution control equipment to the system. Risks posed by the presence of toxic contaminants in the treatment residuals can be mitigated by further treatment for stabilization.

Where practical, on-site incineration can be used to minimize the liability of transporting waste to regional facilities. Unfortunately, the lack of properly trained operators results in incineration being an unsatisfactory alternative for many hospitals.

Off-site regional incineration facilities have some major advantages. Hospitals and other health care facilities do not often have the resources to provide a state-of-the-art system as well as the specially trained personnel to operate it. Advantages offered by regional facilities include the following:

- Financing is often available to obtain a Nuclear Regulatory Commission (NRC) permit allowing incineration of low-level radioactive materials.
- Financing is often available to obtain an EPA Resource Conservation and Recovery Act (RCRA) B permit allowing incineration of small quantities of hazardous waste from hospitals and laboratories.
- Suitable equipment is often available for incineration of large animal carcasses disposed of by medical research facilities.
- Regional facilities can be constructed with duplicate units to minimize downtime.
- A regional facility can afford to have well-trained or certified operators on duty at all times.

Of course, these services are provided to health care facilities at a premium cost, which, in some areas, has risen to such a high level that generators must turn to on-site treatment.

As the most used waste disposal procedure, incineration will be further discussed in detail in Chapter 3.

Incineration is widely recognized as an acceptable means of disposal for infectious wastes, especially difficult-to-handle sharps and pathological wastes. It is conceivable that future regulations may include more stringent standards for operation of infectious waste incinerators. However, one can be certain that this technology will not be disallowed as a treatment/disposal method.

2.3 STEAM STERILIZATION

Steam sterilization is also an oxidation process. In this case, steam is charged into an infectious waste in a pressurized autoclave to kill the bacteria by heat. A large sterilizer is shown in Figure 2.1. This sterilized waste from the sterilizer is subjected to a testing procedure to determine the number of spores that can be incubated. If acceptable, the waste is then ground and/or compacted and disposed of in a landfill. A typical time-temperature curve is shown in Figure 2.2 Sterilization and grinding and/or compaction does not destroy waste. It must eventually be disposed of in a landfill. Currently, many landfills are refusing untreated infectious wastes. It is possible that in the future, even sterilized infectious waste may be refused. Considering the uncertainty over what future regulations may require, it is difficult to predict which types of waste landfills will accept. Some risk is therefore associated with choosing sterilization/compaction since wastes must be ultimately landfilled.

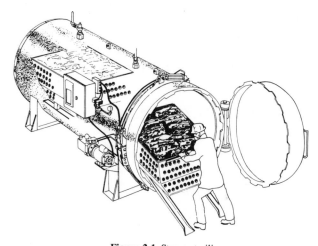

Figure 2.1 Steam sterilizer.

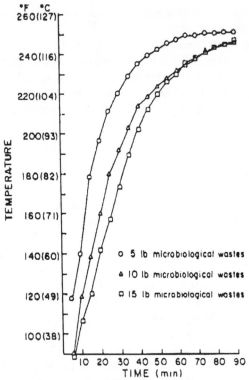

Figure 2.2 Typical sterilization destruction curve [2].

In order to achieve effective and efficient treatment through steam sterilization/compaction, it is necessary to maximize exposure of the entire waste quantity to the desired temperature for a sufficient period of time. The desired temperature is effected primarily by steam penetration, and thus, the degree of steam penetration is the critical factor in achieving the desired effect. Any condition that may prevent proper steam penetration to the waste will diminish the effectiveness of a steam sterilization treatment system.

These limiting conditions include the following:

(1) Use of heat resistant waste containers
(2) Presence of residual air within the sterilizer chamber
(3) Use of deep containers
(4) Failure to open bags and loosen container lids, bottle caps, and stoppers
(5) Loading of the system beyond capacity
(6) Uneven distribution of waste within the sterilization chamber

In addition, any failure of equipment seals or valves resulting in a steam leak may decrease the temperature of the sterilizer chamber and also decrease the effectiveness of the system.

There are some wastes that should not be treated through steam sterilization. Body parts, fluid, and large quantities of animal bedding are generally high-density materials. Direct steam penetration to these wastes may be difficult to achieve. Incineration is recommended for the treatment and disposal of these materials. Antineoplastic drugs (used in chemotherapy), toxic or radioactive chemicals, or any other chemicals that could be volatilized by steam should not be treated through steam sterilization. If sharps are not to be treated, care should be taken to prevent unnecessary tubing, solution bags, and other plastic items from inhibiting steam penetration to the sharps. Incineration is often the preferred treatment method for sharps.

In order to ensure system effectiveness, a steam sterilization process should be monitored and all equipment should be routinely inspected. A testing program, including periodic placement of biological indicators (spore strips) throughout the waste load, is the best method of ensuring proper system performance. *The United States Pharmacopeia* [3] recommends *bacillus stearothermophilus* as a biological indicator for steam sterilization.

2.4 RADIATION

Radiation of bulk materials and medical applications using radionuclides have been used for some time. Now biological materials are being subjected to similar treatment. Radiation sources, such as cobalt-60, at source strengths of 100,000 curies are being considered.

The OSHA exposure rate for biological (pathological) materials is a maximum of 2.5×10^6 R/h (Roentgen per hour) (see Figure 2.3).

There is not, however, any agreement on what required level of radioactivity should be considered standard or sufficient.

Prototype sterilization systems designed by Amerisham Corporation using radioactive sources of 50,000 to 100,000 curies produced dosages of one to two megarads, which was considered adequate [4]. At the current demand rate and production cost, the investment for equipment and shielded room for this type of facility would run from $500,000 to $1,000,000.

Nordion International (formerly Atomic Energy of Canada) for many years has considered the use of radiation sterilization for waste from ships, aircraft, and medical facilities, although other than some pilot programs for disinfection of waste water, they are not aware of anyone using this technique [5]. However, based on the growing scarcity of landfill area and

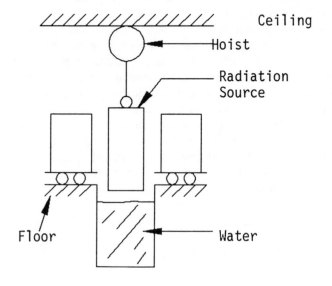

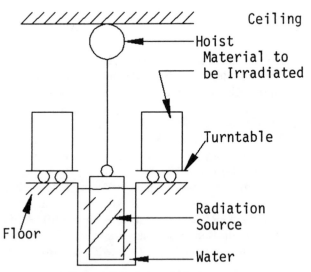

Figure 2.3 Radiation of infectious waste.

concerns over incinerator pollution, they believe that radioactivity has become a very viable waste treatment alternative.

Using their local (Ottawa) costs of $35/ton for landfill disposal and $0.65/pound (including transportation to site) for incineration, Nordion International estimates that, for hospitals generating over seven tons of waste per day, it would be more economical to radioactively sterilize, macerate, and compact for landfill dumping than to incinerate [1]. The economics improve in areas like New York City where landfill costs run around $250/ton [1].

The irradiated waste itself has been reported to be non-toxic. This process and its necessary controls are to be further investigated by Nordion, and in addition, they have commissioned a study by Dr. James Whitby, a member of the University of Western Ontario, to determine (by April 1990) what dosage of radioactivity would be required for the sterilization of different types of waste. Dr. Whitby currently estimates that 3 megarads seem reasonable for sterilization of hospital waste. Others believe that a level as high as 6 megarads would be required for garbage from international transportation, which may be considered dirtier than hospital waste [5].

For a system delivering a three megarad dose and capable of processing 50 tons of waste per day (24-hour operation), the capital cost may be estimated to be in the neighborhod of 3 million dollars for the shielded facility, automatic conveyor and handling equipment, and storage building, not including the cost of the land (approximately 3 acres required).

2.5 MICROWAVING

Microwaving is another technique now being proposed for applications in the United States by a division of Combustion Engineering. In this area, waste is irradiated with microwave energy to disinfect material.

One process, the automatically controlled Sanitec Microwave Disinfection System (see Figure 2.4), starts with refuse being dumped from a hopper to a refuse crusher. The weight of the refuse charge is electronically determined as part of the hopper-filling sequence. Steam conveyed into the filling hopper aids circulation as well as disinfects the crusher chamber. A water mist is injected into the chamber to bind the dust particles. Refuse falls from the hopper into the crushing chamber, and the crushed material flows onto a screw conveyor below. Crushing reduces the material volume by about eight times its original volume. As the material is conveyed, it passes between several banks of microwave coils that are controlled by temperature sensors. The successive microwave banks are activated in stages as required to assure that temperatures of 134°C are reached in each

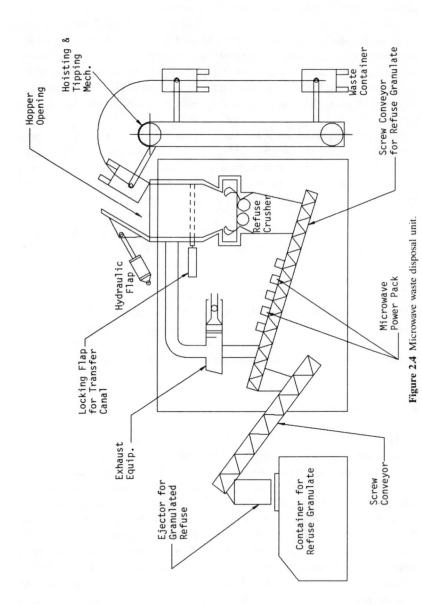

Figure 2.4 Microwave waste disposal unit.

conveyed container. A high-output submicron particulate air filter system removes steam and germs from the air being exhausted from the chamber and at the same time creates low pressure to remove aerosols, steam, and dust particles from the filling hopper. As filters are replaced, the spent filter is crushed and disinfected. Residual fluids from the crushed material are drawn off and evaporated by the microwave energy. The disinfected crushed material is removed from the Sanitec chamber by another screw conveyor and deposited in a refuse container for disposal. Along each processing step, various monitors and control devices assure safe operation and complete sterilization.

The complete Sanitec installation requires a 20 x 26 ft floor space, 11 ft working height, and weighs 8500 lbs. It can handle between 330 to 550 pounds of refuse/hour, operating at a 65 db noise level. Total power consumption is approximately 65 kW per hour [6]. This system is said to use less energy than other disinfection systems, and is environmentally acceptable. A mobile version of this system is available to service small volume laboratories, etc. by travelling to each location to perform disinfection that reduces the risks of transportation of otherwise hazardous waste through the streets.

2.6 HYDROPULPING

Hydropulping, like incineration and sterilization, is also an oxidation technique, and wet pulpers have been developed for the destruction of valuable documents and secret papers. This process can be applied to hospital wastes and can provide for the complete consolidation of most of the wastes by misting the wastes with a liquefying agent during the shredding operation. Pulping systems have an additional advantage in that they can provide for fluidized transport, as well as reduce the waste volume. A typical hospital installation would provide pulping equipment at various locations throughout the building or complex, with a central liquid extractor system being used to remove moisture from the pulped waste before it is conveyed to the refuse disposal site. Pulpable hospital wastes prepared in this matter have a water content of approximately 80 percent, with an attendant increase in weight; however, the resultant waste volume can be as little as 30 percent of the original volume (see Figures 2.5 and 2.6).

The use of pulping systems for general hospital waste is highly controversial. Experience has revealed a difficulty in pulping plastics and cloth. Broken glass and metal grindings have caused severe equipment and plumbing wear. Separation of wastes by the pulpers has not always been successful, and equipment failure was common. However, tangible progress in overcoming these problems is evident in the field. Cutter designs

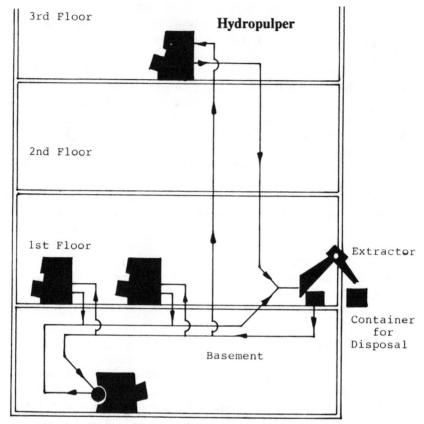

Figure 2.5 Flow diagram of a pulping system for hospital nursing floor waste.

have overcome the problem of pulping plastics and most cloth, although a heavy floor mop may still cause trouble. Improved separators are now being included to remove glass chips, thus reducing equipment and plumbing wear. New materials and heavier designs have improved the reliability of the equipment, and pulpers can now be fed directly by a chute system. A schematic of this type of system is shown in Figure 2.6.

Nevertheless, the use of pulpers for general waste still has serious limitations. It is necessary to segregate all materials that cannot be pulped before they enter the pulping system. This step must be done principally to reduce equipment maintenance problems. Separation before pulping means additional handling at the source of the waste generation, and additional handling is required at the pulper rejection point. Separation of hospital wastes is generally an unsatisfactory requirement not only for the manpower required but also for the health hazards created. Any system that reduces or eliminates sorting is better than a system that does not.

Even with all the recent improvements in the operational features of pulping systems, equipment wear is still greater than desirable. Until pulping systems are capable of handling unsorted hospital waste completely, the use of pulping for general waste is not recommended.

Food service waste, however, may be pulped. This includes food preparation wastes, some packaging materials, tray scrapings, paper and plastic plates, containers, trays, and plastic utensils. Water extractors can remove enough of the water so that the pulp can be incinerated when mixed with other waste in proper proportions or can be dumped with other waste into a compactor for final disposition. In severe low-temperature areas, it may be necessary to protect the slurry and pulp from freezing, and this can be accomplished automatically by a temperature control within the pulpholding area.

2.7 DISPOSAL AND COMPACTION

Compaction is a process that typically produces a four to five times reduction in the waste volume. EPA guidelines discourage the use of compaction alone, although a compactor is a simple device. Large compactors have been used for many years for reducing the volume of infectious and general waste from hospitals. The waste is put into a chamber and a ram then takes the waste and compacts it against a wall. The unit reduces the

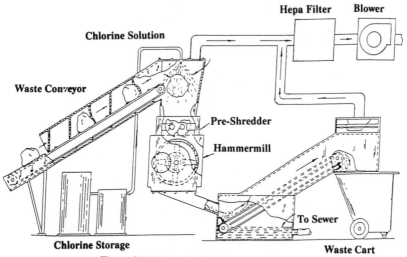

Figure 2.6 Schematic of a hydropulping system.

volume of the waste. There are several floor compactors now being designed and operated at hospitals to make small bales of waste that can then be either landfilled or taken to a municipal or regional infectious waste incinerator for further processing. Generally, in these smaller units, an impervious container is used to hold the compacted waste. The container may then be sealed and shipped for further processing.

The major advantage of this technology is in the volume reduction and improved public perception of the waste. The safety of dealing with infectious waste is also improved in the handling of the containers at a landfill or a municipal incinerator. One of the advantages of the compactor is that there is a tremendous volume reduction (up to 60 percent) in the size of the infected waste but no reduction in weight.

Because the compaction process does not sterilize the material, it is necessary to sterilize the material prior to compaction or to sterilize or incinerate it after compaction. Sending unsterilized waste off-site for processing is not a good practice and has large potential liability problems.

2.8 TREATMENT TECHNIQUES FOR THE FUTURE

2.8.1 STERILIZER/SHREDDER UNIT

The most interesting future technique investigated is the *sterilizer/shredder unit*. To date, this technique has not been tested or marketed commercially, but offers some special benefits including the following:

- potentially lower treatment costs than other techniques (needs to be demonstrated to obtain actual numbers)
- sterilization with reliable biological monitoring techniques available
- volume reduction and a change in the appearance of the waste, possibly making it more acceptable to public scrutiny
- acceptable material for landfill or for further treatment by incineration

2.8.2 DESTRUCTIVE DISTILLATION

Technology is available in which the waste can be thermally distilled to produce gaseous products that can be burned to make steam and to generate electricity. In the process, the waste volume is reduced by 90 percent, and the weight reduced by 75 percent. There is no oxygen in the retort where the gasification process takes place so the waste itself does not burn.

The conditions that produce dioxin and other toxic substances in an incinerator are not present.

The "char", along with the other residue, is sterilized by the heat. Most heavy metals are held in a benign suspension within the carbon. Potentially hazardous materials are chemically converted into clean-burning gases. This procedure has not been tried on hospital waste but is a possible candidate.

2.9 SUMMARY

Oxidation by incineration is currently the most acceptable method for treating infectious waste. Steam sterilization is the other commonly used procedure. In addition, there are four currently used procedures (radiation, hydropulping, oxidation, and microwaving) and three technologies (grinding after sterilization, direct irradiation and distillation) being developed. When costs are included at this time, incineration has the most advantages if the technique is properly utilized. A major advantage is that it provides the greatest volume and weight reduction (approximately 90 and 80 percent, respectively) for this type of waste.

These procedures can all produce a treated waste product that is no longer infectious. However, this may not be the end of the task as the waste residue must still be disposed of in an environmentally safe and aesthetically acceptable manner. It must be checked for RCRA hazard and toxicity potentials and transported and disposed of according to RCRA and Department of Transportation (DOT) regulations.

REFERENCES

1 Cross, F. L. "Comparison of Disposal Technologies for Infectious Wastes," *Proceedings of the Infectious Waste Disposal Conference, Executive Enterprises, Inc. Washington, D.C., October 13, 1988.*

2 Rutala, W., et al. "Decontamination of Microbial Waste by Steam Sterilization," *Applied Environmental Microbiology*, 33 (1982).

3 United States Pharmacopeial Convention. "Sterilization" in *The United States Pharmacopeia*, 19th revision. Rockville, MD:United States Pharmacopeia Convention, Inc., pp. 709–714 (1975).

4 Personal communication with Amerisham Corporation.

5 Personal communication with Nordion International Inc.

6 Peronsal communication with Sanitec Corporation.

Infectious Waste Incineration

3.1 HOSPITAL WASTE

SOLID wastes that are generated at a hospital include paper, plastic, cardboard, food wastes, needles, plus miscellaneous materials that amount to 17–23 lb/bed/day. The amount of waste generated may be approximated from the number of beds in the facility and the occupancy rate. Table 3.1 is a breakdown of the types and quantities of wastes produced by a typical hospital facility.

The size of the incinerator and the amount of energy recoverable from the waste is dependent upon the waste generation rates (pounds/week), the heat content of the waste, the number of hours of operation per day, and the number of days per week that the incinerator will be operating (see Table 3.2 for heat values).

Designers use mass and energy balances to determine the proper size, configuration, and gas volumes/temperatures for a particular incinerator. Waste heat boilers or heat exchangers are often installed after the incinerator to capture the combustion energy from the waste and generate hot air, hot water, or steam.

3.2 PRINCIPLES OF COMBUSTION

3.2.1 THE THREE T's PLUS

In order to ensure good combustion (and this should be a combustion efficiency of 95 percent or better), time, temperature turbulence (3 T's of combustion), and air (oxygen) must be provided.

The Parameter of Time

Residence time refers to the time that the gases remain in the combus-

TABLE 3.1 Waste Types and Quantity.

Type	Wt. % of Total
Pathological	0.5
Infectious	10.0
General	50.0
Food	30.0
Cardboard	9.5
TOTAL	100.0

Note: Average hospital waste amounts to 17–23 lb/bed/day.

tion chambers of the incinerator and is a function of the size of the incinerator, the waste feed rate, and the amount of combustion air.

The Parameter of Temperature

To obtain good combustion, the temperature in the incinerator must be maintained between 1600–1800°F in the first chamber (primary) and 1800–2200°F in the second chamber (secondary).

The Need for Combustion Air

Air (oxygen) is needed to complete the combustion reaction and is typically added in both the primary and secondary combustion chambers. In a controlled air unit, very little air is added to the primary combustion chamber (approximately 15 percent of the combustion air requirements) while as much as 200 percent of excess air is added to the secondary combustion chamber. In a rotary kiln, most of the air (150–300 percent excess air) is added in the kiln (primary combustion chamber) and goes through the entire system with the off gases from the waste combustion.

TABLE 3.2 Hospital Waste Heat Value Approximation.

Waste Type	Wt.%	Btu/lb	Weighted Value
Class 0	70	8,500	5,950
Plastic	15	19,500	2,925
Garbage	10	4,500	450
Class IV	5	1,000	50
		TOTAL (Btu/lb)	9,375

The Parameter of Turbulence

Turbulence is required to mix the burning gases with air to obtain complete combustion. If this is not achieved, then some of the waste organics may go through the unit without total destruction, and this condition is often referred to as stratification of gases in the incinerator. Turbulence is achieved in the incinerator by baffles and by changes in gas direction and burner location.

3.2.2 COMBUSTION

Combustion is a chemical reaction in which oxygen is rapidly combined with a fuel, giving off heat and products of combustion. The oxygen actually combines with the carbon, hydrogen, sulfur, and/or certain other components of the fuel, changing them to different gases. The components of the fuel that aren't burned remain as ash.

The gases that are typically produced are as follows:

$$\begin{aligned}
\text{hydrocarbons} + \text{oxygen} &\rightarrow \text{carbon monoxide and/or carbon di-} \\
&\quad \text{oxide plus water vapor} \\
\text{sulfur} + \text{oxygen} &\rightarrow \text{sulfur dioxide} \\
\text{halogenated compounds} &\rightarrow \text{halogen acids} \\
\text{nitrogen and nitrogen compounds} &\rightarrow \text{nitric oxide, nitrogen dioxide and} \\
&\quad \text{nitrous oxide}
\end{aligned}$$

These gases are chemical compounds in which molecules of each element are combined to produce the compound. When the elements are combined (combustion), heat is given off.

Chemical equations can be used to describe the combustion process. For example, one atom of carbon combines with two atoms of oxygen to produce one molecule of carbon dioxide such that

$$C + O_2 \rightarrow CO_2 + \text{heat}$$

Likewise, two hydrogen atoms combine with one oxygen atom to produce one molecule of water by the reaction

$$2H + O \rightarrow H_2O + \text{heat}$$

Perfect combustion is the result of mixing and burning the exact proportions of fuel and oxygen so that no unburned fuel or oxygen remains.

Often excess air is supplied to the incinerator, but excess oxygen plays no part in the process. For example, if four atoms of oxygen are available to combine with one atom of carbon, two oxygen atoms would be left over.

If not enough oxygen is supplied, all the fuel particles combine with some oxygen but cannot get enough oxygen to burn completely. For example, if two atoms of carbon were combined with two atoms of oxygen, the carbon atoms may share the available oxygen, but neither has enough to become carbon dioxide. Instead they form carbon monoxide (CO), a deadly compound that will form carbon dioxide if more oxygen is provided.

The oxygen needed for combustion normally comes from air. Since air is about 80 percent nitrogen and 20 percent oxygen, the volume of air required for combustion is much larger than the required volume of pure oxygen.

Although the nitrogen in the air does not take part in the combustion reaction, it does absorb some of the heat, which lowers the flame temperature and may form oxides of nitrogen. Thus, the greater the excess air, the greater the temperature reduction.

3.2.3 EXCESS AIR

The fact that excess air tends to reduce the temperature of the combustion process makes it possible to use excess air to control temperatures in the combustion chamber. This, in turn, affects the temperature of the flue gas and the resulting emissions.

Excess air can be determined by an Orsat analysis unit. The method that can be used for an incinerator is as follows.

First an Orsat analysis is done on the plant stack gas during normal operation. Note that the excess air determined at the stack will include leakage, so it is best for the excess air for combustion to be determined at the incinerator gas discharge. The analysis is done either on-site or in the laboratory by analyzing the contents of a plastic bag of gas withdrawn from the stack. The result is the dry gas composition (carbon dioxide, carbon monoxide, oxygen, and nitrogen) by volume.

From the Orsat analysis, the excess air is calculated by the following relationship:

$$\text{percent excess air} = \frac{(\text{percent } N_2) \ (100)}{(\text{percent } N_2) - 3.87 \ (\text{percent } O_2)} - 100$$

where N_2 = nitrogen and O_2 = oxygen.

Example:

Given the following Orsat analysis:

CO_2 =	16%		N_2 =	80%
CO =	0%		O_2 =	4%

Total = 100%

and substituting the values for the percent of nitrogen and oxygen into the equation, the excess air is

$$\frac{(80)\ (100)}{(80)\ -\ (3.87)\ (4)}\ -\ 100\ =\ 24\%$$

The Orsat apparatus is one of the most commonly used gas analyzers. Several types have been developed, all of which are based on the same principles. Basically, the percentage of the main constituents in flue gas are determined by successive absorption of carbon dioxide, oxygen, and carbon monoxide from a measured gas sample in reagent-filled pipettes. The decrease in volume caused by each absorption under constant pressure and temperature is a measure of the quantity of each constituent with the remaining portion of the sample assumed to be nitrogen. The results obtained with each sample are given on a dry basis, and the water vapor present in the flue gas is not usually determined; however, it may be calculated when required to determine the performance or efficiency of the unit.

3.2.4 INCINERATION CRITERIA

A summary of the combustion criteria for infectious waste incinerators is presented below:

PARAMETER	DESIGN/PERFORMANCE CRITERIA
Burnout[1]	≥95%
Combustion Efficiency[2]	≥95%
Primary Chamber Temperature	≥ 1,500°F
Secondary Chamber Temperature	≥ 1,800°F
Secondary Chamber Gas Retention Time	1.0 to 2.0 s

[1]Burnout is a measurement of the residue quality. A burnout of 95 percent means that only 5 percent of the burnable material is left in the residue (ash and noncombustibles).
[2]Combustion efficiency = $[CO_2]/[CO_2 + CO] \times 100$ where $[CO_2]$ is the concentration of carbon dioxide and $[CO]$ is the concentration of carbon monoxide.

3.3 PRIMARY AND SECONDARY COMBUSTION CHAMBERS

Solid waste generally consists of combustibles (volatiles), water, and ash.

Incinerators are designed with one to three chambers to achieve good combustion. Most units, however, have two chambers, a primary and a secondary combustion chamber.

3.3.1 THE PURPOSE OF THE PRIMARY COMBUSTION CHAMBER

The primary combustion chamber (see Figure 3.1) is designed to release the volatile material from the waste and then to continue to burnout any remaining combustible materials from the waste before the ash is removed from the incinerator.

3.3.2 THE PURPOSE OF THE SECONDARY COMBUSTION CHAMBER

The secondary combustion chamber as shown in Figure 3.1 is designed to destroy the volatiles (organics) released from the waste in the primary combustion chamber. The secondary combustion chamber is designed to maintain a 1–2 seconds retention time with temperatures of 1800–2200°F.

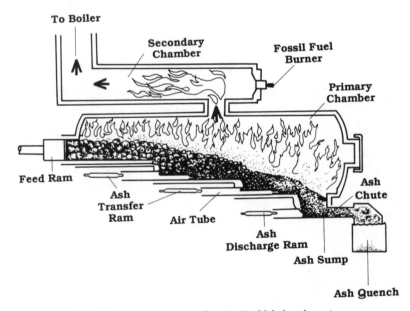

Figure 3.1 Controlled-air incinerator (multiple hearth type).

This ensures that complete destruction of organics takes place and that products of incomplete combustion (PICs) are not formed or go uncombusted through the incinerator.

3.4 TYPES OF INCINERATORS

The two types of incinerators commonly used for infectious waste destruction are the rotary kiln and the controlled air units. Generally, the rotary kilns are used for very large or regional units and the controlled-air types are used by individual hospitals.

3.4.1 ROTARY KILN

A typical rotary kiln incinerator is shown in Figure 3.2. The following lists present the advantages and disadvantages of rotary kilns.

Advantages

(1) Will incinerate a wide variety of liquid and solid wastes
(2) Will incinerate materials passing through a melt phase
(3) Capable of receiving liquids and solids independently or in combination
(4) Feed capability for drums and bulk containers
(5) Adaptable to a wide variety of feed mechanisms
(6) Characterized by high turbulence and air exposure of solid wastes
(7) Continuous ash removal that does not interfere with the waste oxidation
(8) No moving parts inside the kiln
(9) Adaptable for use with many air pollution control devices
(10) Suitable for heat recovery
(11) The retention or residence time of the nonvolatile components can be controlled by adjusting the rotational speed of the kiln
(12) The waste can be fed directly into the kiln without any preparation such as preheating, mixing, etc.
(13) Rotary kilns can be operated at temperatures in excess of 2,500°F making them well suited for the destruction of toxic compounds that are difficult to thermally degrade
(14) The rotational speed control of the kiln also allows a turndown ratio (maximum to minimum operating range) of about 50 percent.

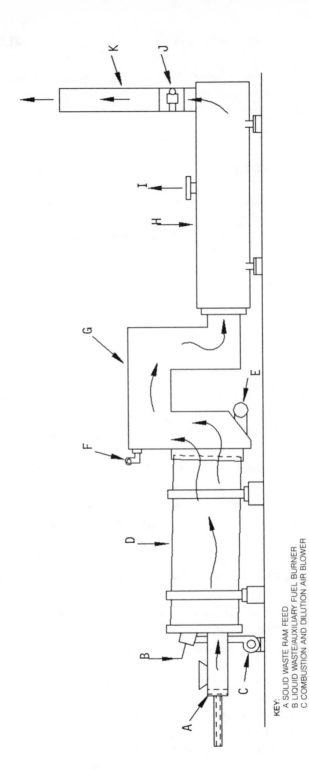

Figure 3.2 Typical rotary kiln incineration system.

KEY:
A SOLID WASTE RAM FEED
B LIQUID WASTE/AUXILIARY FUEL BURNER
C COMBUSTION AND DILUTION AIR BLOWER
D ROTARY KILN INCINERATOR
E ASH DISCHARGE
F LIQUID WASTE/AUXILIARY FUEL BURNER
G AFTERBURNER
H WASTE HEAT RECOVERY BOILER
I STEAM OUTLET
J INDUCED DRAFT FAN
K STACK

Disadvantages

(1) High capital cost
(2) Operating care necessary to prevent refractory damage; thermal shock is a particularly damaging event
(3) Airborne particles may be carried out of kiln before complete combustion
(4) Spherical or cylindrical items may roll through kiln before complete combustion
(5) Frequently requires additional makeup air due to air leakage via the kiln end seals
(6) High particulate loading
(7) Relatively low thermal efficiency
(8) Problems in maintaining seals at either end of the kiln can be significant operating difficulty

3.4.2 CONTROLLED-AIR INCINERATOR

Two types of controlled-air incinerators are shown in Figures 3.1 and 3.3. The following lists the advantages and disadvantages of controlled-air incinerators.

Advantages

(1) Potential for by-product recovery
(2) Reduction of waste volumes without large amounts of supplemental fuel
(3) Thermal efficiency is higher than normal incinerators due to lower quantity of air required.
(4) Reduced uncontrolled air emissions are sometimes possible.
(5) Converts carbonaceous solids into a gas that is more easily combustible
(6) Allows for suppression of particulate emissions
(7) Will burn wastes with a minimum amount of processing
(8) Relatively low capital costs

Disadvantages

(1) May have incomplete burnout of carbonaceous material in ash
(2) Tends to operate on a batch mode because continuous operation may cause problems with clinkers or scale buildup on refractory surfaces

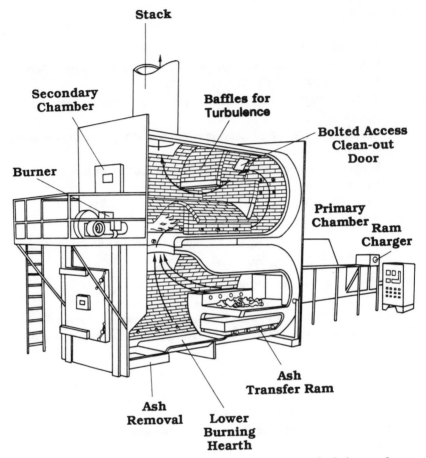

Figure 3.3 Controlled-air incinerator (two hearth type). Courtesy: Atlas Incinerators Inc.

(3) Push plates for ash removal tend to buckle over time
(4) Difficult to control operating parameters when waste stream varies

3.4.3 FLUIDIZED-BED INCINERATOR

A system that could potentially be used is the fluidized-bed system as depicted in Figure 3.4. The major advantages with this design are better heat transfer, better combustion, and less nitrogen oxide emissions because it operates at lower temperatures. The circulating bed unit is shown, but a bubbling bed could also be used. The main disadvantage is that the bed material must be ground to a relatively uniform, small size.

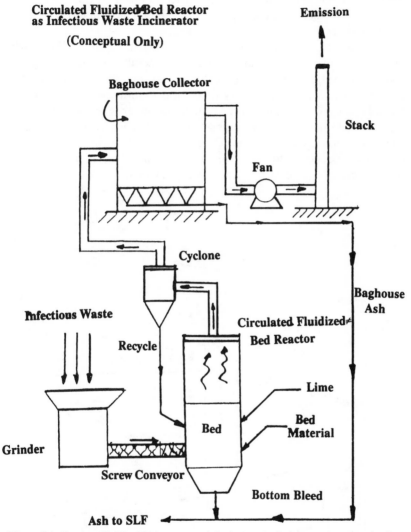

Figure 3.4 Circulated fluidized-bed reactor as infectious waste incinerator (conceptual only).

3.5 INCINERATOR SYSTEM COMPONENTS

An infectious waste incinerator is a combustion device that is designed, built, and operated to render hospital waste(s) innocuous (i.e., render into benign ash and noncombustibles). Ideally, all organic emissions would be reduced to carbon dioxide and water vapor.

A typical hospital incineration system is shown in Figure 3.5. Most manufacturers of the controlled-air incinerators generally use the same type of equipment. Solid wastes are injected (ram fed) into the primary combustion chamber, where the primary function is to turn the wastes into combustible gases. Combustion in the primary chamber releases volatiles that are carried to the secondary combustion chamber where additional air is added for complete combustion. Construction of the primary combustion chamber is essentially the same for all of the manufacturers. In most cases, the incinerator is a refractory-lined steel container.

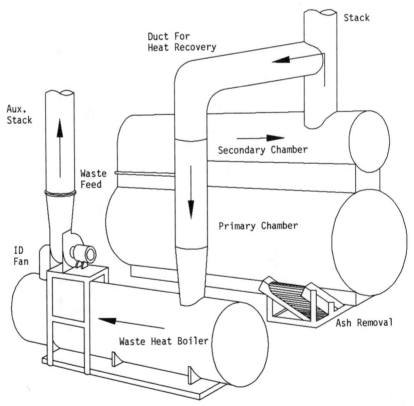

Figure 3.5 Typical hospital incinerator system.

Wastes are injected into the primary combustion chamber in essentially identical fashion by all equipment manufacturers. The automatic sequence of operations includes opening a guillotine door to the chamber, movement of wastes into the chamber by a ram, withdrawal of the ram, closing of the guillotine door, and opening the ram hopper for the next load of wastes. Some designs include automatic spraying of wastes remaining in the hopper with water to prevent fires. The configuration of the secondary combustion chamber has a more varied design. Most of the suppliers provide a chamber of perhaps one-fourth to a volume equivalent to that of the primary chamber (to obtain a 1–2 seconds retention time).

Waste heat boilers, used for energy recovery, are identical to fire tube boilers, with the usual variations (single-pass, double-pass, etc.). They may or may not include a burner. Space must be provided for easy access to the boiler tubers because operators report that cleaning the fire tubes weekly is usually required.

The hot flue gases are drawn through the waste heat recovery equipment and the air pollution control equipment (if required) by an induced draft (ID) fan.

Ash removal from the incinerator depends on the manufacturer and/or model chosen. Some of the incinerators are designed for 24-hour continuous operation, and consequently have continuous ash removal as part of the basic design. Some units are built for batch operation with daily shutdown for manual or automatic ash removal.

Some manufacturers provide a "wet" ash removal system in which ashes are dropped into a sump filled with water; others spray the wastes before dropping them into an ash container. The quenching-type ash removal system is recommended as shown in Figure 3.6, although a mechanical hoe is generally better than a conveyor.

3.6 INCINERATION REGULATIONS

The regulations for infection waste incineration are changing rapidly, and emission levels are becoming more restrictive. These changes mean that burnout must increase. A summary of some state regulations is given in Table 3.3 Combustion efficiency, operator training, and waste ash disposal are also important concerns.

3.7 INCINERATOR SYSTEM COSTS

Controlled-air incinerators are less expensive to install than rotary kiln systems (see Figure 3.7).

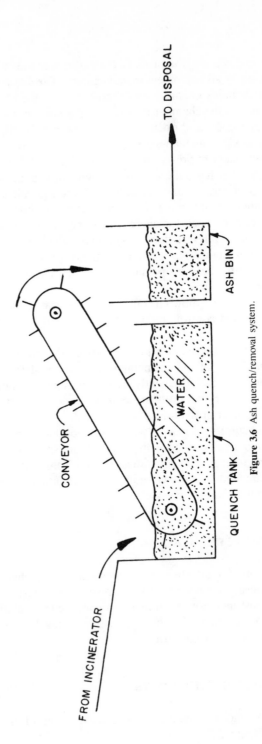

Figure 3.6 Ash quench/removal system.

48

TABLE 3.3 Status of Infectious Waste Incinerator Regulations.

State/Parameter	Indiana	New York	Pennsylvania (500–2000 lb/h)	Alabama (<50 tons/day)	Minnesota (<1000 lb/h)	Mississippi	California	Wisconsin
Air Emissions								
Particulates	0.3 lb/1000 lb DG	.015 gr/dscf[1] at 7% O_2	.03 gr/dscf at 7% O_2	.02 lb/00 100 lb feed	.01 gr/dscf	.2 gr/dscf at 12% CO_2	0.1 gr/dscf	.03 gr/dscf at 12% CO_2
Visible Emissions (Opacity)	—	Hourly avg. 10% max.cont. 6 min. avg. < 20%	30%	20%	—	40%	20%	5% (as measured by U.S. EPA Method 9)
HCl (acid gas)	—	Less restrictive 90% HCl reduction or 50 ppm HCl	30 ppm	—	Testing	—	—	50 ppm at 12%
SO_2	—	50 ppm	30 ppm	—	—	—	—	CO_2 over any continuous 1 hour period

(continued)

49

TABLE 3.3 (Continued).

State/Parameter	Indiana	New York	Pennsylvania	Alabama	Minnesota	Mississippi	California	Wisconsin
Combustion								
Efficiency	—	—	—	—	—	—	—	—
Carbon Monoxide	—	Hourly Average no more than 100 ppm at 7% O_2	100 ppmv	—	—	—	—	50 ppm at 12%
Operator Training								
Training	—	YES	—	—	—	—	—	YES
Certificate	—	YES	—	—	—	—	—	???
Solid Waste								
Residual Burn Out	—	—	On Case by Case basis	—	—	—	—	Max. ash content 5%. No visible unburned combustibles.

[1]Dry standard cubic feet.

50

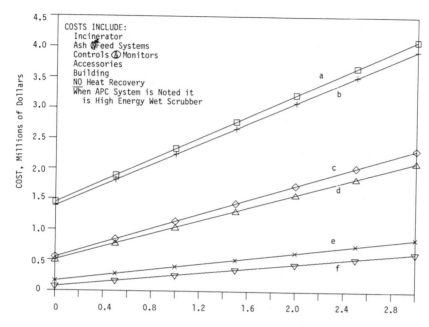

Figure 3.7 Incinerator capital and operating costs for rotary kiln and controlled-air systems in 1988 dollars.

The costs of a controlled-air incinerator include:

- feed system (ram feeder)
- automatic cart dumper
- continuous ash removal
- combustion unit (primary and secondary)
- burners (primary and secondary)
- fan and stack

3.8 REFRACTORY CONSIDERATIONS

3.8.1 GENERAL

Refractory requirements for incinerators vary widely. Refractory selection is governed by five factors, i.e., chemical content, slag, heat, thermal shock, and corrosion, that will be discussed in more detail later. The refractory must be able to withstand occasional temperature excursions considerably higher than the design operating temperature.

The refractory material must be compatible with any slag likely to form on it. The nature of the potential slag formation, including the acidity, major chemical components (iron, heavy metals, alkalies, etc.), and the melting temperature of the slag, must be known.

The presence of chlorine or fluorine will eliminate the use of castable refractories, since these elements will destroy the lime (CaO) binder.

Thermal shock is a rapid change in temperature caused by start-ups and shutdowns, increased feed rates, and runaway reactions.

Corrosion of the steel shell behind the refractory can also be a problem. Many corrosive elements can penetrate the refractory without damage and condense on the shell. However, three ways will be discussed to help protect against corrosion of the steel shell.

3.8.2 REFRACTORY TYPES

Refractories suitable for service incinerators can be divided into three general types: brick, castable, and plastic. Each is different and has its own unique advantages and disadvantages.

Brick refractories are power pressed or extruded into standard or special shapes. They are fired in the refractory manufacturer's plant to develop their strength. The incinerator can be placed in service as soon as the bricks are laid.

Castable refractories are mixed with water like concrete and poured (or cast) into the desired shape inside the incinerator. In large incinerators, they can be applied by pneumatic (gunning) methods that are normally much faster than pouring. They develop their strength from a chemical reaction between a lime-based binder and the water. Castable linings must be dried out before they are placed in service.

Plastic refractories come in a moist, moldable (plastic) form. Unlike castables, no water is added. They are installed in place inside the incinerator by ramming them with special air hammers. They develop their strength when they are fired prior to being placed in service.

3.8.3 CHEMICAL, THERMAL, AND CORROSION PROBLEMS

Refractory requirements for incinerators vary as much as their designs. There is no such thing as a universal refractor recommendation for incinerators; what works well in one incinerator may be completely unsatisfactory in another.

Any refractory selection is limited by five factors: heat, slag, chlorine (or fluorine), thermal shock, and corrosion. A refractor must be compatible with all of these limitations.

All refractory installed in an incinerator should be able to withstand the maximum temperature inside the unit. Almost all incinerators are subject to runaway temperature excursions, and this value should be the limiting temperature, not the routine operating temperature. Also, remember that the effectiveness of any refractory is lowered by reducing atmospheres, slags, hydrogen, and corrosive gases.

The refractory material should be selected so that it is compatible with any slag likely to form on it. It must be known whether the slag is acidic or basic, what the major components are (particularly iron, other heavy metals, alkalies, etc.), the melting temperature of the slag and any other information that can be obtained.

The presence of chlorine or fluorine will eliminate the use of castable refractories. These elements will attack the lime (CaO) binder and destroy it and can cause refractory failures even at very low temperatures.

Thermal shock is a problem for most incinerators. This is a rapid change in temperature caused by start-ups and shutdowns, increased feed rates, runaway reactions, and other causes. Some refractories can be severely damaged in short periods of time by rapid temperature changes while others are much more resistant to rapid temperature change.

Corrosion of the steel shell behind the refractory may have a major input on refractory selection and design. Many corrosive elements can penetrate the refractory without damaging the refractory and condense on the shell causing serious corrosion. A good refractory design and material selection can reduce or eliminate this problem. There are three ways to protect against corrosion with refractory linings:

(1) The refractory lining can be designed so that it will conduct enough heat to the shell to keep the shell temperature above the dew point of anything likely to condense on it. This is perhaps the best way to protect against corrosion; however, it results in considerable heat loss and can be a hazard to workers in the area.

(2) An acid resistant lining can be placed between the shell and the refractory. These acid resistant linings must be selected and installed with great care.

(3) Very dense refractories with low porosity can sometimes reduce or eliminate penetration by corrosive components of the atmosphere inside the incinerator.

3.8.4 REFRACTORY SELECTION

Brick

Advantages

(1) High density and low porosity; better resistance to slag penetration

(2) Ceramic bonding; greater strength and resistance to destructive forces in their temperature range

(3) Good hot strength in some types of brick

Disadvantages

(1) More subject to damage by thermal shock than other types of refractory

(2) Slag attack and penetration at the joints

(3) Cost; generally brick is the most costly refractory because of the extra labor required to install it.

Recommendations

(1) Lower temperatures and no slag problem—high duty or super duty

(2) Low temperature and slag—high-fired super duty

(3) Moderate temperatures and moderate slag—high-alumina brick such as 70 percent alumina

(4) High temperature and severe slag—mullite-bonded or alumina-chromia

These are just general recommendations. Specific recommendations may vary considerably from the general guidelines. It is advisable to consult the refractor manufacturer before making your decision.

Castables

Advantages:

(1) The easiest and cheapest to install of all refractories

(2) Good resistance to thermal shock

(3) Some dense castables have good resistance to slag

Disadvantages

(1) They lack the strength and slag resistance of brick and plastics

(2) Castable linings must be pre-fired or heated very slowly on the initial start-up

(3) Binders can be destroyed by chlorine or fluorine.

Recommendations

(1) Low temperature and mild slag—super duty castables

(2) Moderate temperature, moderate slag—high-alumina castables
(3) Moderate temperature, severe slag—chrome-based castables
(4) Higher temperature—very high alumina castables

Plastics

Advantages:

(1) Excellent resistances to thermal shock (as a group, better than brick or castables)
(2) Good slag resistance
(3) Generally good compromise in properties between brick and castables

Disadvantages:

(1) Must be fired-in before placing the incinerator in service

Recommendations:

(1) Lower temperature and moderate slag—super duty
(2) Lower temperature and severe slag—phosphate-bonded plastic
(3) Higher temperature and moderate slag—high-alumina materials
(4) Higher temperature and severe slag—high-alumina phosphate-bonded or alumina–chromia phosphate-bonded

This presentation is intended to provide general information only. Before selecting a refractory lining for your incinerator, please contact a refractory manufacturer to discuss your particular application.

3.8.5 INSTALLATION TIME

Installation time varies greatly with the size and complexity of the unit. The following is a rough relative comparison of installation times for different types of refractories (starting with the fastest):

(1) *Castables (gunned)*—This is normally the fastest means of installing a refractory lining. The castables are blown through a hose under pressure and mixed with water at the nozzle and sprayed onto the surface. This can work only for vessels large enough for someone to get into them with the equipment and do the gunning. More material is required for this application because refractory particles bounce off the surface (rebound) and do not stick. Rebound losses require an additional 10 to 25 percent more material.
(2) *Castables (poured)*—Pouring castables like concrete behind forms is

normally the second fastest way to line an incinerator. If complex forms are required, ramming plastics may be faster.

(3) *Plastics*—Ramming plastics with special air hammers is normally somewhat slower than pouring castables. Again, the size and complexity of the unit determines the time investment.

(4) *Brick*—Brick normally takes the longest time to install. Special cutting and fitting required by unusual surfaces can greatly extend this time. The advantage to the brick lining is that it can be placed in service as soon as it is installed, whereas castables and plastic must be fired-in.

The purpose of firing-in the castables is to drive out the water. There are many fire-in schedules for refractory castables ranging from 30 to 100°F per hour with designated holding periods of one-half to one hour per inch of thickness.

3.9 SUMMARY

Waste material can be successfully treated in an environmentally acceptable manner in a properly designed and operated incineration system. Under these conditions, 95 percent burnout of the combustible feed material at combustion efficiencies of 99 percent or greater can be expected. The type and quantity of waste will help dictate the type of incineration system that will be best for each particular facility. Other factors, such as regulatory requirements, space, and location in the community will further dictate system type. For example, large and noisy rotary kilns are not good for small community facilities with little space, and systems that use large containers of solid feed are not suited to fluidized beds.

Incineration systems should include emission control equipment. The air pollution control devices help protect against release of halogenated and other acid gases, particulates and vapors (e.g., toxic metals). Other emissions occur during improper ash discharge. Both types of emission controls are necessary for "complete" incineration systems.

Incinerator Control and Operation

4.1 AIR EMISSION CONTROLS

4.1.1 GENERAL TYPES

PROPERLY operated incineration systems may require particulates and/
or gaseous emission controls in order to meet local regulations. These
control devices are often complicated to use properly and are expensive.
Table 4.1 lists five control devices commonly used. A facility installing
an incinerator at this time should consider the installation of air pollution
control equipment now or allow space for adding this equipment as it
becomes a requirement in the future.

Figure 4.1 is a schematic of an incineration system showing feed/ash/
particulate matter feed rates. In this figure, example quantities of particulates are listed for this system. Note that control of gaseous emissions may
also be required in which case the system may look more like the arrangements shown in Figures 4.2 and 4.3.

In a regional facility where either a rotary kiln or controlled-air unit
may be used, a particulate control device will be required to meet many
state regulatory requirements. In addition, because of the chlorinated
plastics, acid gas emissions will need to be controlled with an absorber.
The regulations for infectious waste incinerators are changing rapidly and
becoming more restrictive, and in order to meet the new requirements,
complicated control devices may be required which will cost additional
monies and require rather sophisticated operation.

4.1.2 OPERATION AND MAINTENANCE PROGRAM

There are number of useful reasons for setting up an operation and

TABLE 4.1 Comparison of Air Pollution Control Systems for Infectious Waste Incinerators.

Parameter	Wet/Dry Scrubber	Wet/Wet Scrubber	Venturi/ Packed Tower[1]	Baghouse Packed Tower	Calvert Scrubber
Efficiency	99.9%	99.9%	99%	99.9%	99%
Particulate	0.015 gr/dscf	0.015 gr/dscf	0.03[1] gr/dscf	0.01 gr/dscf	0.03 gr/scf
HCl	85%	75%	98%	98%	98% (100 ppm)
	No Visible Plume	No Visible Plume	Visible Plume	Visible Plume	Minimum Visible Plume
Space Requirements	40' × 60'	40' × 60'	20' × 40'	30' × 40'	30' × 40'
Wet/Dry Systems	Wet	Dry	Wet	Dry/Wet	Wet
Residuals Generated	Wet	Dry	Wet	Dry (baghouse) Wet (packed tower)	Wet
Treatment Chemicals	Limestone Solution	Dry Limestone	Liquid NaOH or Lime Solution	Liquid NaOH or Lime Solution	Liquid NaOH or Lime Solution
Required Ancillary Equipment	• Lime Storage • Mixer	• Lime Storage	• Chemical Storage • Clarifier • WWT	• Chemical Storage • Clarifier • WWT	• Chemical Storage • Clarifier • WWT

[1]Venturi Scrubber/Packed Towers will typically achieve 0.03 gr/dscf at a pressure drop across the venturi of approximately 30″ water column.
WWT—Waste Water Treatment

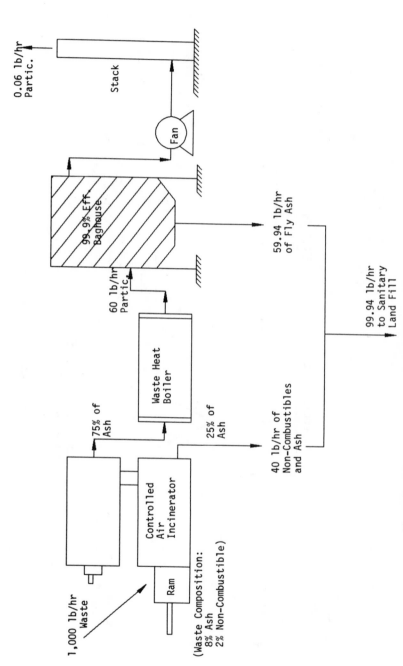

Figure 4.1 Feed/ash/particulate matter mass flow rates for infectious waste incinerator.

0.06 lb/hr
Partic.

Stack

Fan

99.9% Eff
Baghouse

60 lb/hr
Partic.

59.94 lb/hr
of Fly Ash

Waste Heat
Boiler

75% of
Ash

25% of
Ash

99.94 lb/hr
to Sanitary
Land Fill

40 lb/hr of
Non-Combustibles
and Ash

Controlled
Air
Incinerator

Ram

1,000 lb/hr
Waste

(Waste Composition:
8% Ash
2% Non-Combustible)

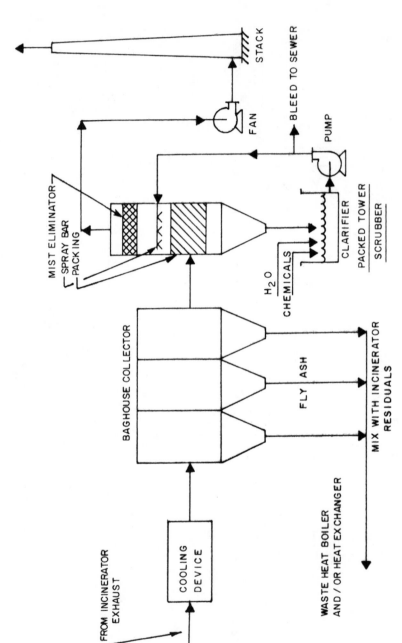

Figure 4.2 Baghouse/packed tower air pollution control system.

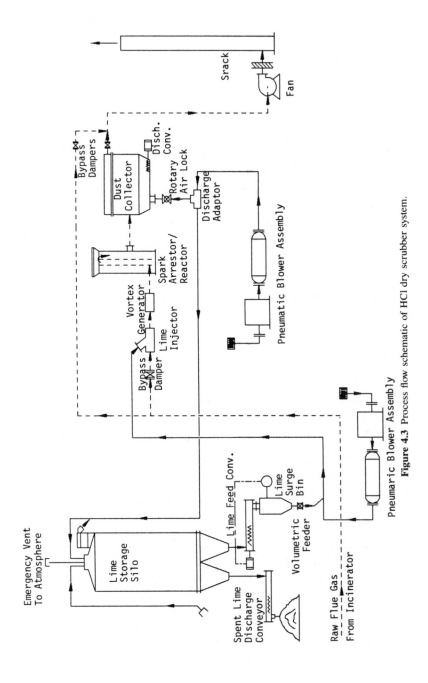

Figure 4.3 Process flow schematic of HCl dry scrubber system.

61

maintenance program. Some of the advantages of this type of program are as follows:

- early detection of malfunctions
- predict failures and thereby prevent them
- identify and correct problems as they occur
- prevent damage to equipment
- reduce air pollution emissions (improve product recovery)

Management should also be interested in the benefits of such a program, which may include the following:

- reduced operating costs by requiring less operator time, power, fuel, services, equipment replacement and parts inventory
- compliance with emission regulations/standards
- extending the life of control equipment
- recovery of valuable products

Items often overlooked in the design stage are features necessary to carry out proper operation and maintenance and may include the following:

- adequate access openings
- test ports
- static pressure taps
- platforms and stairs
- adequate instrumentation to monitor equipment operation
- alert systems to warn operations personnel of impending malfunctions

Since many key inspection points may be impossible or impractical to instrument, it is important to have a schedule for frequent and complete external and internal inspections of the equipment.

The general inspection principles involved are as follows:

(1) Design
- selection of appropriate equipment
- understand the functions of the various parts
- system controls and auxiliary components
- access to equipment to perform inspections

(2) Operational
- knowledge of equipment operating principles
- start-up and shutdown procedures
- equipment adjustments and operation
- routine surveillance
- maintaining operating records

(3) Maintenance
  - lubrication
  - equipment inspections (internal and external)
  - prompt adjustments, repairs, and replacement of parts
  - general sight and sound during operation

(4) Optimization

(5) Safety

All air pollution control systems generally consist of the following:

  - process
  - duct system
  - prime mover
  - control device(s)
  - stack

The control device itself may require no inputs if it is a purely mechanical collector, or it may require the input of energy, usually in the form of electricity or fuel and/or steam, and may require dry and/or liquid chemicals. In many systems, there will be a product, by-product, or waste to remove.

Some of the parameters that should be considered in the routine operation of the system are as follows:

(1) Production rate

(2) Fuel and raw material

(3) System gas flow rate
  - calibrated flow measurement equipment
  - induced draft (ID) fan power input

(4) System resistance(s) (pressure drop)
  - ID fan static pressure
  - collector resistance(s)
  - duct and stack resistances

(5) Stack gas characteristics
  - temperature(s)
  - gas composition
  - moisture content
  - others, depending upon process (e.g., particle size and size distribution, corrosive potential, etc.)

(6) Control equipment function indicators

(7) Ancillary equipment function indicators

Routine operation and maintenance also includes the emission monitoring system(s). Some of the items that should be included are as follows:

(1) Monitoring particulate emissions
   - mass emission sensors (Beta gage, etc.)
   - dust catch rate (material collected in hoppers, clarifiers, etc.)
   - plume opacity and appearance
(2) Monitoring gaseous emissions
   - mass emission sensors
   - chemical usage for absorption systems
   - fuel analysis
   - raw material analysis

Maintenance serves to safeguard against breakdowns by detecting potential problems and eliminating them. Preventative maintenance is better and cheaper than repairs after breakdown and also serves to keep production moving. Preventative maintenance includes maintenance planning schedules, establishing priorities, system organization, and control cost checking. Some of the items that should be part of a system maintenance inspection for air pollution control systems are listed below.

(1) Air infiltration
   - process equipment
   - breaching and ducts
   - access doors and panels
   - expansion joints
(2) Induced draft fan
   - vibration
   - bearing temperature
   - bearing lubrication
   - coupling lubrication
   - V-belt condition
   - motor bearing lubrication
   - foundation bolts
   - variable speed drive
(3) Thermal insulation
   - integrity
   - cold spots
(4) Dampers
   - functions
   - lubrication
(5) Temperature elements
   - thermocouples
   - pyrometers
   - hot wires

(6) Pressure sensors
   • traps and lines
   • transmitters

One of the areas often overlooked is the start-up and shutdown of the control equipment. Internal and external inspections may be to no avail if the start-up and shutdown procedures are not followed very carefully. For example, during start-up, a dry collector may have to be heated and pass through a dew point temperature zone. On shutdown, the control equipment could again pass through this temperature zone. In this system, warm moist gases should be purged before cooling in order to prevent or minimize ash buildup and/or corrosion problems. An alternative to this procedure is to always keep the system warmed above the dew point.

Some general thoughts related to start-up and shutdown of typical dry and wet systems are listed below. For details on specific equipment, refer to the appropriate chapter.

Start-Up and Shutdown Procedures for Dry Collectors

(1) Start-up of equipment
   • Has the collector been cleaned out?
   • Are access hatches tightly closed?
   • Start-up and check out the dust removal system.
   • Start the induced draft fan and preheat the system.
   • Start the process.
(2) Shutdown of equipment
   • Empty hoppers before stopping process.
   • Stop the process.
   • Purge the system with air.
   • Stop the fan.
   • Check to ensure hoppers are empty.
   • Have the system cleaned out.

Wet collectors do not have dew point problems but have other problems (e.g., abrasion and chemical attack such as erosion and corrosion) and tend to be more sensitive to start-up and shutdown problems than dry collectors.

Start-Up and Shutdown Procedures for Wet Collectors

(1) Start-up of equipment
   • Check that the scrubber and associated equipment are cleaned out.

- Close all access openings.
- Start the system pumps.
- Start the chemical treatment system.
- Start the sludge removal system.
- Start the induced draft fan.
- Start the process.

(2) Shutdown of equipment
- Stop the process.
- Stop the induced draft fan.
- Purge the liquid systems.
- Turn off the chemical feeders to the waste treatment system.
- Stop the pumps.
- Purge the sludge removal system.
- Make sure that the scrubber is clean.
- Make sure that the sludge removal system is clean.

4.1.3 WET SCRUBBERS

Most scrubber problems, assuming the proper unit has been selected for the given application, involve spray nozzle plugging, liquid circuit restrictions, and entrainment of droplets from the vessel. Other less common problems are outlined below. An example of a wet scrubbing system is shown in Figure 4.4.

Wet/Dry Line Buildup

Improper scrubber design allows a dry dust-laden gas to contact the juncture of the scrubbing liquid and the vessel, causing dust buildup. Good designs prevent this contact by extending ductwork sections sufficiently into the scrubber and thoroughly wetting all scrubber surfaces through reliable means (usually a gravity flush and sometimes sprays).

Nozzle Plugging

Nozzles plug through improper selection such as too small orifices through which too dense scrubbing liquid must pass, improper header design, drawing off a sump that also settles (and concentrates) solids, erratic pump operation, chemical scaling, and mechanical failure.

Flow Imbalance

The headers external to the scrubber are very important because they must send the manufacturer's required flow to the proper location at the

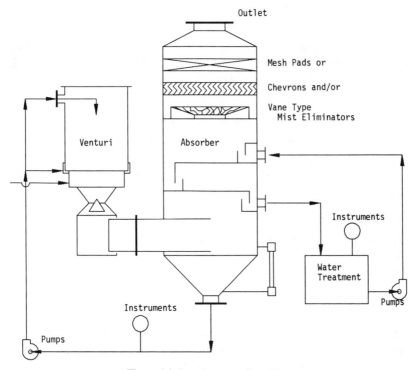

Figure 4.4 Quencher venturi scrubber.

proper rate. Many problems are solved through simple flow adjustments using the existing valves.

Buildup (Scaling)

Scaling is the plating out of deposits on a scrubber surface and is usually harmless unless the surface in question is a functional one. It is caused by the chemical composition, solubility, temperature, and pH of the scrubbing liquid. It is a difficult problem to diagnose, but a good deal of research has been done on calcium-based SO_2 scrubber scaling problems. Proper control starts with the scrubber design and process control.

Localized Corrosion

Corrosion is a major factor in shortening the operating life of a scrubber whether properly designed or not. Wells or pockets of liquid should be avoided and points of stress should be adequately flushed. Internal members attacked from two sides should be thicker than the shell.

Instrumentation Fitting Blockage

One problem that is a significant cause of problems is instrumentation blockage. Many times a standard fitting is not adequate in a scrubber and specially designed fittings and connections must be used.

Sump Swirling

Especially on cyclonic devices, the swirling of the scrubbing liquid can cause severe wear and drainage problems unless arrested by anti-swirl plates in the scrubber or rapid continuous draining.

Entrainment

Entrainment occurs when the droplet separator is not functioning properly. Nearly all scrubbers produce entrainment, but only the good ones eliminate it prior to discharge.

Reentrainment

Reentrainment occurs beyond the droplet removal device through improper draining or erratic flow patterns. It can also occur in stacks of very high velocity or where fittings protrude into the high-velocity air area.

Liquid–Gas Maldistribution

The gas and liquid must be properly distributed for the given application. Each affects the other, as maldistribution can be aggravated by the influence of baffles (needed or accidental), buildup, mechanical failure, wear, scaling in headers, or improper design. This is most common in packed and spray towers.

Thermal Shock

When hot gas meets a cold scrubber something has to give. Proper design permits gradual cooling rather than abrupt changes. Typically, a simple problem to fix through the use of multiple cooling zones, thermal shock is sometimes discovered only too late.

Loss of Seal

All scrubbers run in variation to atmospheric or ambient conditions. The juncture of the liquid circuit with its surroundings is oftentimes a liquid seal. This seal may be at the top of a quencher or on an overflow connection. These lines must have seals capable of preventing gas movement to or from the ambient surroundings. Loss of seal can cause entrainment or plugging and instrumentation malfunction.

Wear

Wear can be tolerated unless it is localized. Unfortunately, a scrubber's functioning parts are also the ones that wear. Expect to replace fun wheels if they are constantly sprayed with water as in dynamic scrubbers, venturi throats on venturi scrubbers, and any other high-velocity zone. Remember, gases take the path of least resistance (not necessarily the shortest path). When checking for wear, be suspicious of those parts that inhibit this flow (parts directly along the path of least resistance).

Vibration

Vibration is most common in wet dynamic scrubbers and with the fans in wet fan venturi or cyclonic systems. It is best controlled by monitoring and scheduled preventative maintenance.

4.1.4 ABSORBERS

Absorbers are wet scrubbers specifically used for controlling gaseous emissions. Table 4.2 is a summarized trouble-shooting checklist for a packed tower absorber.

TABLE 4.2 Packed Tower Absorber Problems/Solutions.

Problem	Possible Solutions
Poor Gas Distribution	1. Use an injection-type support grid. 2. Allow extra vertical height inlet to grid. 3. Use less than 8 ft/s vertical velocity.
Poor Liquid Distribution	1. Install redistributors every 4–6 ft of packing. 2. Rearrange headers and liquid entry. 3. Use a reflux distributor grid.
Packing Sized Improperly	1. Check with packing manufactuer not scrubber designer. (Many companies ignore recommendations.)
Velocity Too High	1. Put another tower in parallel with existing unit. 2. Cut back in flow rate if possible.
Velocity	1. Restrict bottom part of grid. 2. Use small packing. 3. Use redistributors. 4. Raise water level.

4.1.5 BAGHOUSES

Baghouses or fabric filters are the most efficient particle collecting devices when designed, installed, and operated properly. They require periodic maintenance, spare parts, and a knowledge of the entire system. Table 4.3 and 4.4 present a sample maintenance schedule and spare parts inventory, respectively, while Appendix 1 is a troubleshooting guide to baghouse air pollution control systems.

4.2 INCINERATOR OPERATION

In the past, poor operating practices have resulted in excessive air emissions, including acid gas emissions, odors, particulate fallout, and visible emissions. These emissions have been the result of overcharging the unit, inadequate temperatures, poor adjustment of air, and poor design. Because of this, many states, including New York, Indiana, Massachusetts, California, Pennsylvania, and Wisconsin, have enacted regulations or have draft legislation requiring training for hospital incinerator operators.

Operators of incinerators must be familiar with the entire system, not with just the incinerator. Great detail has been provided in the previous section on emission control equipment, and this section will present information on the incinerator and some of its connection hardware (e.g., fans, dampers, and valves).

4.2.1 ROUTINE OPERATION

Incinerator operational procedures must be established for each system and must be tailored to each specific installation with its peculiar problems because every installation can be different. The procedures must be taught to the operators and a check method must be initiated to ensure that the procedures are followed. The following is a general guide to incinerator operations.

Routine Start-up

(1) Examine the unit carefully. Make sure it is clean, that the doors and interlocks operate properly, that it is purged of all combustible/explosive vapors, that both the primary and secondary burners ignite and burn cleanly, and that temperature and pressure instruments are set at the recommended set points.

(2) Close all doors, start fans and purge with air for two minutes or longer if the temperature is $>300°F$.

TABLE 4.3 Periodic Maintenance Schedule for Baghouses.

Daily
1. Check pressure drop.
2. Observe stack (visual or with opacity meter).
3. Walk through system listening for proper operation (audible leaks, proper fan and motor functions, bag cleaning system, etc.).
4. Note any unusual occurrences in the process being ventilated.
5. Observe all indicators on control panel.
6. Check compressed air pressure.
7. Assure that dust is being removed from the system.

Weekly
1. Inspect screw conveyor bearings for lubrication (do not over lubricate).
2. Check packing glands.
3. Operate all damper valves (isolation, bypass, etc.).
4. Check compressed air lines, including line oilers and filters.
5. Check bag cleaning sequence to see that all valves are opening and closing properly.
6. Spot check bat tension (inside bag collectors).
7. (High-temperature applications) Verify accuracy of temperature-indicating equipment.
8. Check pressure drop indicating equipment for plugged lines.

Monthly
1. (Shaker) Check all shaker mechanism moving parts.
2. Inspect fan(s) for corrosion and material buildup.
3. Check all drive belts and chains for wear and tension.
4. Inspect and lubricate appropriate items.
5. Spot check for bag leaks.
6. Check all hoses and clamps.
7. Check accuracy of all indicating equipment.
8. Inspect housing for corrosion.

Quarterly
1. Inspect baffle plate for wear.
2. Thoroughly inspect bags.
3. Check duct for dust buildup.
4. Observe damper valves for proper seating.
5. Check gaskets on all doors.
6. Inspect paint.
7. Check screw conveyor flighting.

Annual
1. Check all bolts.
2. Check welds.
3. Inspect hopper for wear.

TABLE 4.4 Spare Parts[1] Needed for Baghouse Operation.

- bags
- bag support cages (reverse pulse and plenum pulse)
- bag clamps
- seals and caulking material
- solenoids
- diaphragms
- timer components
- baffle plates or wear plate sections for baffle
- bat connecting rods (shaker and reverse flow)
- tensioning springs (reverse flow)
- belts for shaker mechanism (shaker)
- motor for shaker mechanism (shaker)
- fan belts
- spare bearings and gasketeing for all mechanical components

[1]Quantities of parts will vary as to manufacturer's suggestions and the type of process.

(3) Ignite the main burner and bring up the temperature of the primary chamber to its recommended level over the recommended heating rate compatible with the refractory limitations.

(4) Charge with 50 percent of the normal waste charge.

(5) Ignite secondary burner and adjust for clean stack.

(6) Adjust air flow to recommended value and begin normal operation when specified temperatures are achieved.

Routine Operation

(1) Charge at periodic intervals in accordance with operating instructions. Weight or volume measurements ±5 percent will ensure good incinerator operation provided the density of the charge is consistent.

(2) Adjust air flow and temperature of afterburner chamber to achieve clean stack (visual). Excess air flow should be reduced to an absolute minimum (or recommended value if measurement equipment is available) and the afterburner should be maintained at a minimum fuel level to produce a clean stack.

(3) Continue charging at the recommended rate, but decrease the rate if an increase in unburned waste develops in the incinerator.

Routine Shutdown

(1) Stop incinerator feed.

(2) Determine that the charge has been incinerated and only ash remains.

(3) Shut down main ignition or support burner if still operative.

(4) Shut down secondary burner and cool at the rate recommended for the refractory used.

(5) Purge with air until the temperature is reduced to 300°F.

(6) Shut off blower and see that all interlocks are secured. If draft is induced, leave the blower in operation.

(7) Open charging and access doors and shut off induced draft blower.

Normal Burning Period

A two-stage unit, when burning normally, will run with the lower burner off and also with the upper burner off or at a low-fire position. The flameport and the underfire air valve will be modulating. Temperatures will range in the upper chamber from 1700 to 2150°F and in the lower chamber from 1400 to 1700°F.

If there are underfire air tubes, they should be rodded out periodically (every four hours). If the ash is removed by an ash hoe, it should operate every 20 to 30 minutes.

If feed is removed by an internal ram, it should operate every 15 to 20 minutes and stroke one-third of the full stroke capacity.

4.2.2 UPSET CONDITIONS

The unit may occasionally have an upset. Some of the visible signs of upset are unit smoking, lower chamber temperature too low or too high, unburned material in the ash, and constant feed ram recycling if the unit is so equipped. Each of these conditions will be addressed in detail.

Unit Emitting Black Smoke

Black smoke indicates unburned gases and can be caused by low upper chamber temperature, lower chamber draft too high, feed material content too high, or material too high in Btu content, and may also be produced if the main burner failed or is not operating properly, the flameport air blower is not modulating or off, or if the linkage on the flameport air or underfire air slipped. Upon observing black smoke, an operator should check the following:

(1) Main burner

(2) Flameport air

(3) Underfire air (draft in the lower chamber)

(4) Feed rate (material Btu)

To stop the unit from smoking black, place the feed system in manual and raise the charging door off of its lower limit switch. This will cause the flameport air valve to open fully. Close the underfire air valve then raise the setpoint on the main burner.

Unit Emitting White Smoke

White smoke indicates too much air in the upper chamber or particulate ash from the lower chamber. Upon observing white smoke, an operator should check for the following:

(1) flameport air valve linkage

(2) lower chamber draft

(3) underfire air linkage

(4) main burner

To stop white smoke, the operator should close the flameport air valve, close the underfire air valve, increase the feed rate, and check to see if a large pile of ashes has built up in the rear of the lower chamber.

Lower Chamber Temperature Too Low or Too High

If the temperature is too low, the cause could be due to a rapid feed rate or low-Btu value material that prevents the underfire air from penetrating the pile. Upon noticing a reduced chamber temperature, an operator should check the following:

(1) The underfire air linkage

(2) The feed rate (decrease or stop feeding material)

(3) The underfire air ports (rod if necessary)

If temperatures are too high, the cause may be due to a slow feed rate, too much underfire air, a broken water seal on the ash pit, or a gap at the bottom of the charging door. Upon observing an elevated chamber temperature, an operator should check the following:

(1) Underfire air linkage

(2) Water level in ash pit

(3) Charging door (close if necessary)

(4) Feed rate (increase to raise the temperature)

Upset Conditions—Unburned Material

This condition is usually caused by a too rapid feed rate cycling of the internal ram or from stroking the internal ram too far. If unburned material is observed in the ash, an operator should check for the following:

(1) The feed rate (slow down if necessary)
(2) The interval timing of the internal ram (increase as needed)
(3) The forward stroke on the internal ram (decrease as needed)

4.2.3 FEED RATE

The feed rate is determined by the unit size, the heat content (Btu) of the material being burned and local, state, and federal air quality regulations. The following is an example of the feed rate determination for a unit with a 13,000,000 Btu/h capacity:

Assume that a 6,000,000-Btu burner normally operates at 20 percent capacity. This burner can then produce

$$20\% \text{ of } 6,000,000 = 1,200,000 \text{ Btu/h}$$

This unit's total capacity is 13,000,000 Btu/h, so its waste feed capacity becomes

$$13,000,000 - 1,200,000 = 11,800,000 \text{ Btu/h}$$

For example, because of its high plastic content, a certain waste is rated at 8500 Btu/lb. The feed rate for this unit would then become

$$\frac{11,800,000 \text{ Btu/h}}{8500 \text{ Btu/lb}} = 1388 \text{ lb/h of infectious waste}$$

So an operator can charge the unit with 138 lb of waste every 6 minutes or alternatively, 231 lbs every 10 minutes.

4.2.4 BURNERS

Much has already been noted about burners. They are used for refractory curing, start-up, and for supplemental heat if necessary. Gas and oil are the most common types. Table 4.5 lists possible flame problems that could occur in an oil burner and techniques for troubleshooting their cause.

The three basic burners for incinerators are the following:

(1) Gas Burners
(2) Oil Burners
(3) Combination Gas–Oil Burners

TABLE 4.5 Oil Burner Troubleshooting Summary.

Flame Problem	Possible Cause	Areas to Check
Flame away from burner	Too much primary air	Primary air shutter, Linkage, Fan
Smokey flame	Not enough air	Oil pressure, Cup position
Flame too long	Too much oil, Incorrect cup position	Oil valves, Burner cup
Flame too wide	Too little primary air, Incorrect cup position	Primary air shutter, Linkage fan, Burner cup
Sparky flame	Oversized bits of oil and carbon	Cup (clean, possible adjustment)
Pulsating flame	Oil amount incorrect, Uneven oil flow, Too little air	Oil temperature, Oil pressure, Air supplies

Each of these types can be divided into many sub-types that are classified by various configurations such as mixing, draft arrangement, and atomizing systems.

Gas Burners

The types of gas burners can be divided into three basic categories:

(1) *Raw Gas Burners.* The raw gas burner is one in which the gas is introduced into the combustion air as a pure fuel at the point of ignition. This type is usually used when there is a high level of excess air supplied either by a natural or a forced draft system.

(2) *Nozzle Mix Burners.* The nozzle mix burner is essentially a raw gas burner except that mixing with air occurs at the end of a single injection nozzle within the burner. Air–fuel ratios are controlled as compared with a raw gas burner that doesn't attempt to control the air–fuel ratio. The nozzle mix burner usually employs mechanically liked valves or dampers to control this ratio, but may also use a "zero" regulator arrangement.

(3) *Premix Burners.* The premix burner takes several forms. The true premix burner generates a fuel–air mixture and pipes it to one or more burners. This system is usually used for multiple burners where a constant ratio is required on each of the burners. A major shortcoming of this type of burner is the potential for flame flashback from the point of ignition to the point where the mixture is first generated. It is not widely used due to this problem.

Oil Burners

There are many designs, modifications, and patents on oil burners. The simplest method of classifying them is on the basis of the method by which the fuel is made combustible (i.e., changed from a liquid that won't burn into a vapor or mist that will burn). Before describing the various oil burner classifications, the basic components of an oil burner should be analyzed.

The first part is the liquid injector. The liquid must be transported into the furnace or combustion chamber and it must be either finely divided, atomized or vaporized.

Atomization can be accomplished by forcing the liquid through a small opening (oil fire) under air pressure, by spinning the oil in a cup or on a disc at a high rate so that it sprays off into the burner, or by combining the oil with a stream of compressed air.

The second part of the burner or combustor is the windbox. The windbox is the point at which air is introduced into the burner body and usually contains a vane fan. Burners may be forced draft or natural draft depending upon the type of system into which they are firing. Forced draft burners are inherently more efficient and better combustors because they can achieve higher air velocities than natural draft systems. The natural draft units are dependent upon the height of the stack, and therefore, the pressure drop is quite critical.

The third part of the burner is the combustion chamber. Most commercial burners utilize the downstream device into which they are firing as the combustion chamber and have only a refractory flame burner block or tile that supports the base of the flame.

Oil burners, therefore, can be divided into several categories either by the type of mixing or by the type of atomization. The first classification, the type of mixing, is either forced draft or natural draft. The type of atomization can be either mechanical, low pressure air, high pressure air, steam, or sonic, and the mechanical atomization includes the rotary-cup-type of unit.

Combination Gas–Oil Burners

Combination burners permit the use of either gas or oil as a fuel. The use of combination burners makes it possible to take advantage of the economic breakpoint between gas and oil at various seasons of the year and/or through price fluctuations of the two fuels. The combination burner, while more expensive initially, can offer significant savings during operation.

The combination burner is essentially an oil burner with the necessary adaption to permit firing of natural gas or liquid petroleum. This additional equipment usually involves a nozzle mix type of burner with arrangements as described previously.

Ignition Systems

Most burners are spark ignited. This process involves a spark plug similar in many ways to what might be found in the standard automobile except that the industrial spark plug has a higher voltage and a wider gap. The voltage normally employed for industrial burners is in the range of 6,000 volts.

An ignition transformer converts 120-volt input power to 10,000-volt secondary coil output.

Burner Controls and Safety Equipment

The safety equipment that is required on either an air, gas, or combination system is fairly closely specified by the major insuring agencies (e.g., Factory Manual, which gives a list of approved components and also specifies certain arrangements that are acceptable or unacceptable).

Generally, these safety regulations involve the following:

(1) That the entire system, depending upon its downstream volume, be purged with air for a certain period before ignition of the gas pilot or main burner ignition. This is to ensure that no combustible mixture exists within the incinerator

(2) That there be a limited trial for ignition of the pilot after which it will be necessary to go back to a pre-purge condition for the entire system

(3) That the main burner ignites within a specified time period, usually in seconds, after the main fuel valve has been opened

(4) That an approved flame failure device be utilized on the burner

Flame Failure Devices

Flame failure devices can be separated into three groups:

(1) Flame rectification devices (flame rod)

(2) Photo cells

(3) Photochemical active cells

Auxiliary Equipment

In addition to the items described in the control system for burners, such things as combustion air blowers for forced draft burners, normally called turbo blowers, are used to supply air to the system. Most forced draft burners utilize 100 percent primary combustion air that must be supplied by fans or blowers.

Fuel oil pumps are normally of the gear-pump-type achieving pressures from 30–400 psig. The pressure is controlled by a relief valve on the discharge side of the pump, which recirculates some of the fuel back to a storage reservoir.

Burner Fuel Consumption

The next section will present information with examples on how to check your incinerator burners. This check is intended for burners using fuel oil, natural gas, and butane.

The advantage of these checks are as follows:

(1) To reduce costs by optimizing fuel consumption
(2) To reduce volatile organic compound (VOC) emissions for burners running over capacity (rich mixture)

4.2.5 MAINTENANCE AND TROUBLESHOOTING

Information summarized here is relative to various system components. In addition, see also the specific sections on Air and Gas Flow (4.2.11), Burners (4.2.4), and Refractory Considerations (3.8).

Typical Maintenance Problems

To continue to obtain reliable service from your incineration equipment, it is necessary to perform periodic inspections and maintenance servicing.

TABLE 4.6 Incinerator Maintenance Schedule.

Component	Maintenance	Frequency
Ultraviolet flame detectors (burners)	Clean lens	Monthly
Opacity Monitor	Clean light source and receiver lens	Monthly
Fan	Grease bearings	Semiannually
Burners	Clean spark plugs	Semiannually
Combustion Chamber	Check refractory for damage	Annually
Damper Motor	Lubricate	Annually
Fan	Clean Blades	Annually

Table 4.6 summarizes some of the typical maintenance tasks necessary to operate an incinerator. Detailed servicing procedures covering these components listed in the table are provided.

Cleaning the Spark Plugs

To clean the spark plugs, remove each spark plug assembly from the base of its respective burner. Clean the tip of the spark plug electrode and its grounding point using fine steel wool or fine sandpaper. Be sure to remove any soot or carbon buildup. After cleaning the spark plug assembly, reset the spark plug gap (the distance between the electrode and ground point) according to the specifications provided with the equipment.

Cleaning the Flame Detectors

To clean the flame detectors, remove the device from the base of the burner by loosening the nut that attaches the flame detector to the burner plate nipple. Locate the lens inside at the end with the attachment nut. Clean this lens with a dry cotton cloth or tissue, removing any soot or carbon buildup. After cleaning, replace the detector on the burner pipe nipple by hand tightening the nut. (Do not use a wrench.)

Fan Motor Lubrication

The fan motor must be lubricated occasionally. Locate the grease fittings on the motor and lubricate using an all-purpose grease.

Cleaning the Fan

The fan should be cleaned annually to ensure that proper movement of air in and around the incineration equipment is maintained. To remove the fan for cleaning, disconnect the electrical power, remove the fan from its mounting, and visually inspect the fan blades. Dirt buildup on the blades should be scraped off. Do not remove small balance weights located on some blades.

Burner Gas Adjustments

The burner gas settings for each burner should be checked annually and adjusted separately and may be done by reading the fuel consumption with the burners running. Proper gas firing rates are very important to pollution-free operation, extended life of the refractory, and fuel conservation. To change the firing rate, adjust the manual gas valve on each burner.

This procedure should be attempted only by a skilled, trained technician or a gas company representative.

Refractory Inspection

The refractory in the incinerator should be inspected and evaluated annually. Prior to entering the incineration equipment, be sure that gas and electrical services are turned off and have another person outside the incineration equipment to ensure that the utilities are not accidentally turned on while the inspection is in progress.

Inspect the refractory in the combustion chamber, flameport, inside the main loading door, and in the secondary combustion chamber. Make sure that the refractory has not fallen away, exposing any of the steel structure. The refractory in these areas should be a minimum of 4½ inches thick. General wear or spalling of up to a 2-inch depth can be tolerated, but should be noted for future repairs. Wear or spalling beyond a 2-inch depth should be repaired as soon as possible. Consult the equipment vendor or refractory supplier for further instructions.

Fan Maintenance

Table 4.7 lists some of the inspection activities involved in fan maintenance.

Troubleshooting

An incinerator is a relatively simple device, and except for routine maintenance checks, the only areas where troubleshooting may be necessary involve the blower and burner(s). Make sure the power supplies are turned off before performing any service on incineration equipment.

Troubleshooting the Blower

If the blower does not start:
(1) Check the power source of supply breaker.
(2) Reset the motor starter by depressing the start button.

Troubleshooting the Burner

If the burners will not fire:
(1) Check to be sure the safe run light is on.
(2) If the safe run light is on, check the loading door safety switch to be sure the door is in the correct position.

TABLE 4.7 Fan Maintenance Schedule.

Activity	Frequency	Remarks
Grease fan bearings	Semiannually	Use the type of grease suggested by the fan supplier
Check fan for excessive vibration	Daily	Vibration must be minimized immediately
Check fan belts for proper tension or wear	Daily	If belt is loose, tighten immediately; replace if worn or cracked. Be certain to replace with proper size and type of belt (keep spares on hand)
Thoroughly inspect stack for holes, cracks, leaks, etc.	Annually	Repair the stack as soon as practical
Verify fan speed with a tachometer	Semiannually	If speed is off, check for proper belts and sheaves, alignment and belt tension. Changing the belts/ sheaves may be required, or the motor may need replacement.
Have the fan wheel spin balanced	Annually or when repairing	By contract service

(3) Check the air safety switch to be sure the blower is providing sufficient air.

Troubleshooting the Oil Burner

(1) *Flame away from the burner* is most likely caused by the flame being pushed off by too much primary air. Check and clean the air nozzles and/or adjust the primary air according to the manufacturer's instructions.

(2) *A smokey flame* (unstable and flickering) means not enough air. The primary and secondary air controls should be lubricated, cleaned, and reset according to the manufacturer's instructions. Fan blades may need to be cleaned and belts tightened.

(3) *Flame too long* means too much oil is entering the burner. The oil metering valve should be adjusted by the oil company representative.

(4) *Flame too wide* means the air cone around the fuel mixing cup is not strong enough.

(5) *Sparky flame* is caused by a dirty, damaged, or incorrectly positioned fuel mixing cup. If cleaning and adjusting the cup doesn't help, call for service.

(6) *Pulsating flame* (flame changes in rhythm—large, small, large, small, etc.) is generally caused by uneven oil or air flow or not enough air. Check the oil temperature and the air flow pressure for proper adjustment.

Figure 4.5 provides a summary of these burner troubleshooting procedures.

Table 4.8 lists some of the suggested spare parts for an incineration operation. This list is a general compilation only.

4.2.6 MOVING MATERIAL THROUGH THE INCINERATOR

Figure 4.6 shows the common methods of moving waste, ash, and noncombustibles through an infectious waste incinerator. Both batch and continuous type systems are shown.

INCORRECT FLAME	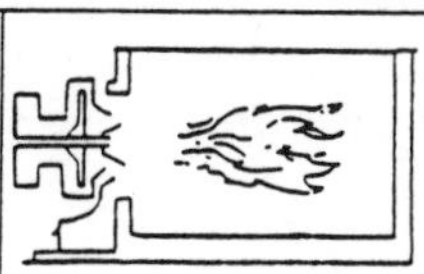	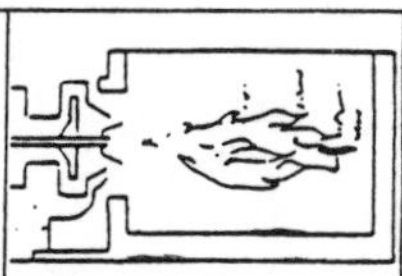	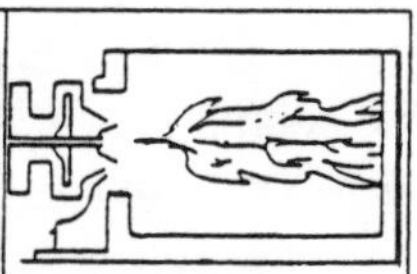
HOW INCORRECT	FLAME AWAY FROM BURNER	SMOKY FLAME	FLAME TOO LONG
POSSIBLE CAUSE	Too much Primary Air	Not enough air	Too much oil Incorrect cup position
CHECKS TO MAKE	Primary Air shutter, linkage, fan	Primary Air shutter, linkage Secondary Air Windbox, linkage Stack Damper	Oil Valves Burner Cup

INCORRECT FLAME	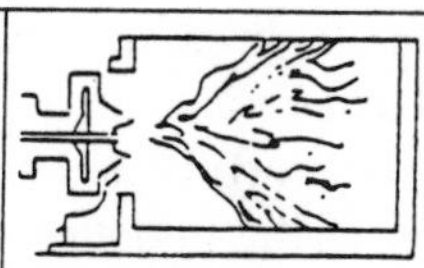	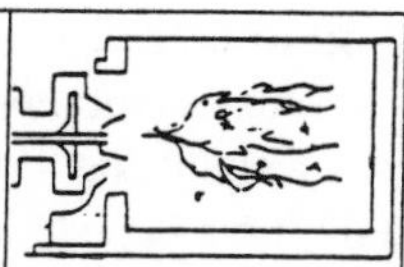	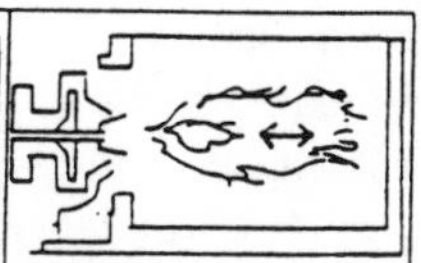
HOW INCORRECT	FLAME TOO WIDE	SPARKY FLAME	PULSATING FLAME
POSSIBLE CAUSE	Too little primary air; Incorrect cup position	Oversized bits of oil and carbon	Oil amount incorrect Uneven oil flow Too little air
CHECKS TO MAKE	Primary Air shutter, linkage, fan Burner Cup	Cup — Clean, possible adjustment	Oil Temperature Oil Pressure Air Supplies

Figure 4.5 Flame troubleshooting guide.

TABLE 4.8 Suggested Spare Parts for an Incinerator.[1]

- hydraulic fluid
- one set of hydraulic cylinder seals for each size supplied
- flame safety relay for burner(s)
- flame sensor(s)
- limit switches or other position indicators
- thermocouple of each type supplied
- temperature controller of each type supplied

[1]Although spare parts depend to a great extent on the individual manufacturer, the above items should certainly be considered where applicable.

4.2.7 ASH HANDLING EQUIPMENT

Figure 4.7 shows three types of ash removal devices that may be used in addition to or in place of ash rams. Typical original quantity and spare parts for one type of ash hoe system are listed in Table 4.9.

4.2.8 CHARGING METHODS

Essentially all hospital waste is fed as solid waste. Solids are fed into an incinerator in three ways: (1) ram feeders or multiple ram feeders, (2) screw-auger feeders, and (3) conveyors. Each one can be modified to provide continuous or batch feeding. Solid feeds are discussed first, then liquid waste feeding.

Ram Feeding System

Ram feed systems are probably the most common type of feed system used with smaller incinerators (up to 50 tons/day). They are designed to limit air infiltration into the primary combustion chamber thus minimizing the potential for a flashback from the incinerator. Ram feeders can handle noncontainerized wastes as well as bags, fibre drums, and boxes. Large bulky items must be removed or reduced in size prior to incineration.

Ram feeders are often designed to operate on an automatic cycle once the feeding process is manually initiated. Waste is loaded into a feed hopper by hand, conveyor, or small loader (Bobcat). Smaller units will have a hopper cover that must be closed prior to the initiation of the feed sequence. Larger units will normally use a series of two or more rams to isolate a portion of the hopper contents before feeding into the combustion chamber.

Figure 4.8 shows the main components of a ram feeder. The automatic sequence of events (see Figure 4.9) for loading a charge into the primary combustion chamber includes opening a guillotine door to the chamber,

(a) BATCH TYPE UNIT
(Burn/Burn Down/Cool/Clean Cycles)

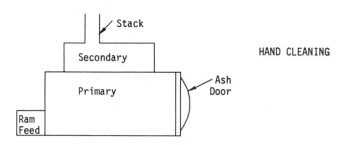

HAND CLEANING

(b) CONTINUOUS UNITS (24 HOURS/DAY)
i. MECHANICAL PLOW

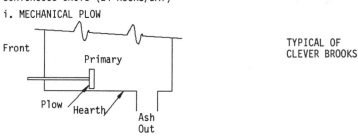

TYPICAL OF
CLEVER BROOKS

ii. PUSH PLATES

TYPICAL OF
SIMMONS, ATLAS,
ECP

iii. PULSE HEARTHS

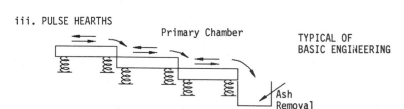

TYPICAL OF
BASIC ENGINEERING

Figure 4.6 Moving material through an incinerator.

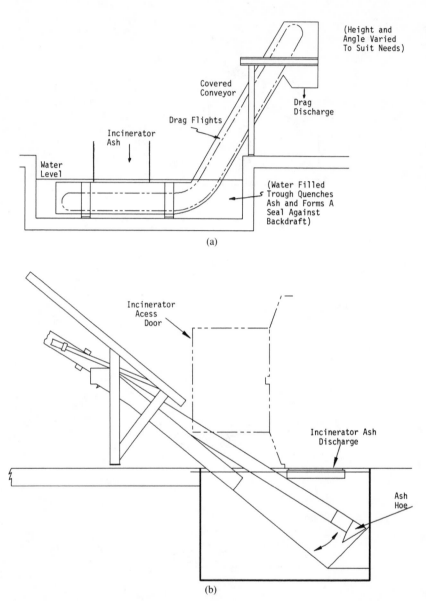

(Height and
Angle Varied
To Suit Needs)

Covered
Conveyor

Drag
Discharge

Drag Flights

Incinerator
Ash

Water
Level

(Water Filled
Trough Quenches
Ash and Forms A
Seal Against
Backdraft)

(a)

Incinerator
Acess
Door

Incinerator Ash
Discharge

Ash
Hoe

(b)

Figure 4.7 Incinerator ash handling devices: (a) Wet bottom ash drag conveyor; (b) Backhoe ash removal system; (c) Wet ash sweep.

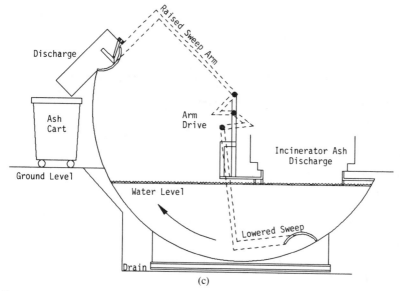

Figure 4.7 (continued). Incinerator ash handling devices: (a) Wet bottom ash drag conveyor; (b) Backhoe ash removal system; (c) Wet ash sweep.

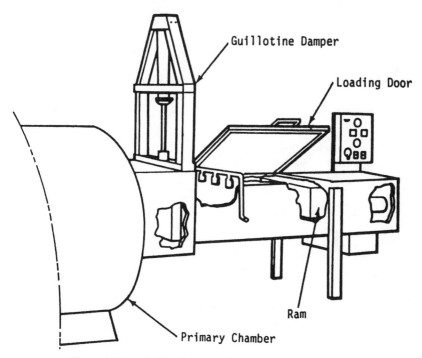

Figure 4.8 Ram feed loading device for controlled-air incinerator.

TABLE 4.9 Typical Spare Parts for Ash Handling Equipment (Ash Hoe Type System).

Item	Quantity	Recommended Spares
Hydraulic Cylinder (Ash Hoe)		
Piston Seal Kit	1	1
Rod Seal Kit	1	1
Rod Brushing Kit	1	0
Hydraulic Cylinder (Hoe Lift)		
Piston Seal Kit	1	1
Rod Seal Kit	1	1
Rod Brushing Kit	1	0
Hydraulic Cylinder (Hoe Carriage)		
Piston Seal Kit	2	1
Rod Seal Kit	2	1
Rod Brushing Kit	2	0
Bearing	1	0
Water Level Probe	1	0
Solenoid Valve	1	0
Water Level Switch	1	0
Roller	4	0
Roller Mount	4	0
Roller Shaft	4	0
Blade	1	0
Bearing	1	0
Hydraulic Hose (5/8 dia)	138 ft.	0
Male Connector (per each size)	5	0
Male Elbow (per each size)	5	0
Union	14	0
Tee Union (per each size)	2	0
Hydraulic Tee (per each size)	3	0
Female Connector	3	0
Hydraulic Tubing (3/8 o.d.)	14 ft	0
Hydraulic Tubing (5/8 o.d.)	46 ft	0
Bulkhead Union	6	0
Port Bushing	5	0
Hex Bushing	2	0
Hollow Hex Plug	6	0
Close Nipple	4	0
Stem	48	0
Ferrule	48	0
Tube Clamp	21	0

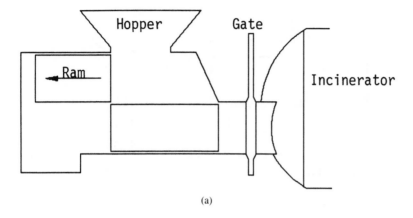

(a)

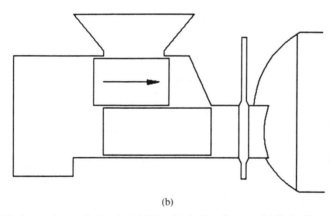

(b)

Figure 4.9 Automatic ram feed cycle: (a) Waste loaded into hopper; (b) Hydraulic ram isolates waste from previous charge; (c) Second ram moves to allow waste to fall into feed chamber; (d) Fire gate opens, ram moves forward, waste pushed into combustor.

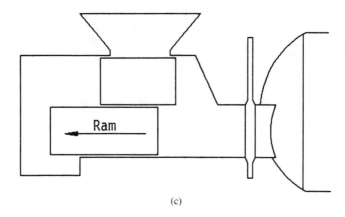

(c)

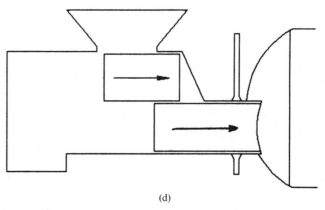

(d)

Figure 4.9 (continued). Automatic ram feed cycle: (a) Waste loaded into hopper; (b) Hydraulic ram isolates waste from previous charge; (c) Second ram moves to allow waste to fall into feed chamber; (d) Fire gate opens, ram moves forward, waste pushed into combustor.

moving the wastes into the chamber by a ram, withdrawing the ram, closing the guillotine door, and then opening the ram hopper for the next load of wastes.

Screw-Auger Type Feeders

Screw feeders are similar to ram feeders in their sequence of feed steps but are better suited to handle noncontainerized waste, however, heavy duty systems can break apart bag boxes and even wood pallets. Screw feeders can provide continuous or batch feeding.

Waste is normally fed into a hopper. The auger in the bottom of the hopper rotates carrying the waste into the combustion chamber. The speed of the auger varies the feed rate and can be computer controlled.

Waste that is normally containerized due to its toxicity is broken up in the auger; consequently, the auger must be regularly decontaminated.

Conveyors

Conveyors are often used in combination with ram or screw type feeders. This type of arrangement offers greater flexibility for feeding different types of wastes.

Liquid Wastes

Liquid fuels must be vaporized before combustion can occur. The degree of atomization and fuel–air mixing is directly related to burning efficiency. Liquid wastes are fed, under 50–150 psi pressure, through small orifices in the nozzles or burners located in the primary or secondary combustion chamber. High pressure steam or air is injected into the spray providing effective atomization. Feed rates vary from 10 to 100 gallons per hour depending on the properties of the liquid.

4.2.9 DRAFT CONTROL

Good draft pressure control of negative 0.03–0.30 inches water column is essential to satisfactory incinerator performance. Large systems provide draft control by using forced draft induced draft fans, while smaller systems with no pollution control devices can use dampers. The cheapest damper system is a counterweighted barometric damper, next a rotary barometric damper, and the most expensive is the hot valve that is installed in the stack or breeching and modulates off of the lower chamber draft reading.

The lower the draft pressure that can be controlled consistently, the bet-

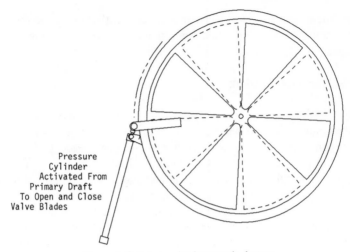

Pressure
Cylinder
Activated From
Primary Draft
To Open and Close
Valve Blades

Figure 4.10 Rotary valve barometric damper.

ter the effectiveness of the incineration process. Barometric dampers can control only from about 0.20–0.30 in H_2O and must be at about 60°F. Rotary barometric dampers are controlled by a valve that operates off the primary chamber draft as shown in Figure 4.10 and can control from 0.10–0.20 in H_2O. Both types add air to the stack. A hot valve in the stack can control from 0.05–0.15 in H_2O water continuously and down to 0.03 in H_2O when required. Dilution and cooling is minimized but the equipment cost is the greatest. This type of damper is like a butterfly valve and is shown in Figure 4.11.

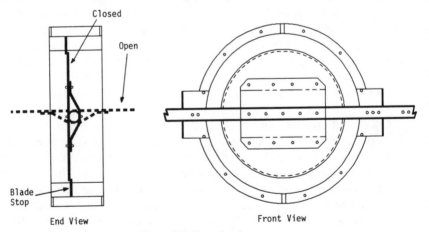

Closed

Open

Blade
Stop

End View   Front View

Figure 4.11 Hot valve damper.

4.2.10 CLINKERS

Clinker problems are the result of excessive temperature in the primary chamber. Most ash residue begins to become soft and tacky at temperatures between 2200–2500°F, depending upon composition. As a result, this material tends to fuse together and form a large, dense mass that can adhere to the hearth areas or prevent mass flow through the incinerator in those units equipped with ash removal systems. The easiest cure for clinker problems is to operate the primary chamber at the lowest temperature possible that is consistent with acceptable carbon burnout and operating regulations. Depending upon the type of underfire air system provided, it is frequently found that clinker formation occurs even though chamber thermocouples indicate proper primary chamber temperatures. The reason for this problem is that most thermocouples indicate the temperature of the gas-filled chamber above the burning refuse bed, as the localized temperatures in the immediate vicinity of individual underfire air ports are usually much higher. In fact, it is not unusual for dazzling yellow-white flame patterns to occur in front of individual air ports that indicate temperatures in excess of 2500°F. Parts of these small flames most likely approach stoichiometric conditions with associated maximum flame temperatures. For this reason, it is usually best to have a larger number of smaller underfire air ports in lieu of a smaller number of larger ports. In this manner, small localized clinkers may form but are not given a chance to adhere to each other and accumulate.

One procedure to prevent clinkers in controlled air incinerators is to take advantage of the water–gas reaction in which hot carbon is contacted with steam to produce carbon monoxide and hydrogen gas. Both of these gases are further combusted in the secondary chamber. The advantages of the carbon–steam reaction is that the reaction is endothermic which results in the minimization of localized hot spots in front of individual underfire air ports and subsequent clinker problems, and additional fixed carbon conversion efficiency is achieved.

4.2.11 AIR AND GAS FLOW

Fans and dampers are used to control the air and gas flow within the incinerator. Since they are an integral part of the incinerator design, a brief review of the various types of fans is presented first.

Fans

A *straight radial blade fan* has four or more blades. It is low in both efficiency and cost, and is generally selected for slower speeds, although it can produce a very large tip speed [see Figure 4.12(a)].

The *forward-curved blade fan* depicted in Figure 4.12(b) may have as many as 40–50 blades. It is generally similar to the straight radial blade fan in efficiency and application. It is somewhat more costly than a straight radial blade fan, but can be operated somewhat out of balance without damage.

The *radial-tipped blade fan* is more efficient than either a straight radial or forward-curved blade fan [see Figure 4.12(c)]. It is often selected as an induced draft fan and may have as many as 32 or 34 blades. This type requires a larger housing than a straight radial and costs more than either a straight blade or a forward-curved radial; however, it is quieter and easier to keep clean since it has a tendency to throw off fly ash. Since the buildup tends to be relatively even, the fan has less tendency to become unbalanced.

The *backward-inclined flat blade fan* shown in Figure 4.12(d) can be used only when the incoming air is clean. Buildup of material at point *A*, for instance, will cause serious imbalance problems that would probably destroy the fan. The fan does, however, have a fairly high efficiency.

The *backward-inclined airfoil blade fan* has a high efficiency and high cost. Eight to ten (or more) airfoil blades may be used as shown in Figure 4.12(e). Although this type of fan is seldom used for induced draft, it is often used for forced draft. Again, the air must be clean for it to function properly.

Forced Draft Fan Systems

A forced draft system is one in which the fan is at the inlet end of the system and blows or forces the air into the system. Forced draft fans have either the backward-inclined, flat-blade wheel, or the backward-inclined, air-foil blade wheel. In general, they have ten to twelve blades.

Induced Draft Fan Systems

An induced draft system is one in which the fan is downstream of the inlet and draws air into the system. When the gas to be handled is unlikely to be clean, the best choice is the radial-tipped fan.

Installation and Maintenance

Fans must be straight and level with all anchor bolts tightened evenly. Most complaints of fan vibration can be traced to improper installation.

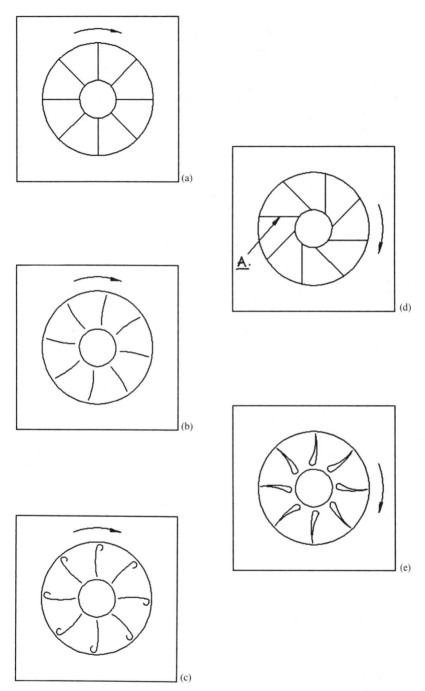

Figure 4.12 Types of fan blades: (a) straight radial blade; (b) forward-curved blade; (c) radial-tipped blade; (d) backward-inclined flat blade; and (e) backward-inclined airfoil blade.

Both forced and induced draft fans must be cleaned as completely as possible, including all blades, to prevent the development of unbalance conditions.

In general, the only other maintenance a fan requires is at the bearings or grease fittings on the dampers and vanes. An inspection and maintenance schedule is provided in Table 4.10. Considerable care should be taken to follow the manufacturer's recommendations on acceptable lubricants. An induced draft fan will require more frequent inspections than forced draft fans due to the nature of their service. Safety glasses should always be utilized for lubricant inspection.

Dampers

The volume of air from a fan can be controlled either by adjusting the fan speed or by dampers. Fan speed control is more effective. Figure 4.13 contains diagrams of three types of dampers. A brief explanation of each follows.

A *parallel blade damper* tends to direct the air to one side of the duct as it closes. It can more or less completely shut off the flow, but it is not as good as a guillotine damper [see Figure 4.13(a)].

TABLE 4.10 Typical Fan Inspection and Preventative Maintenance Schedule.

Inspection/ Maintenance Item	Daily	Weekly	Monthly	Semiannually
Vibration Check	X			
Oil Level		X		
Oil Color		X		
Oil Temperature		X		
Lubricate		X		
Bearings Check				
noise	X			
leaks			X	
cracks			X	
loose fittings			X	
inspection (internal)				X
clearances, wear, pitting, scaring)				
Clean and Inspect Blades				X[1]
and Internal Housing				
Fan Belt				
noise check	X			
belt tension and wear	(check whenever the fan is out of service)			

[1]Fans in scrubber service may require cleaning on a weekly, monthly, or quarterly schedule.

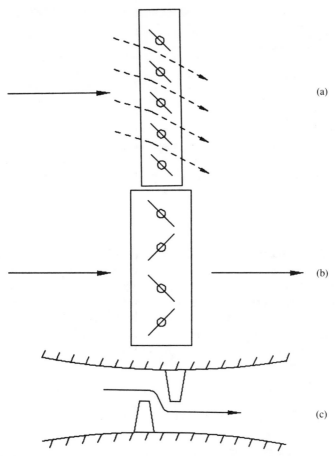

Figure 4.13 Flow control dampers: (a) parallel blade; (b) opposed blade; and (c) inlet valve.

An *opposed blade damper* produces a straight flow that provides equal air distribution downstream of the duct. This type of damper can completely shut off the air flow as shown by Figure 4.13(b).

An *inlet valve* can control (or limit) the flow to approximately 25 percent of the wide-open volume with leakage through the center only [see Figure 4.13(c)].

4.2.12 ENERGY EVALUATION

The combustion process in an incinerator can be evaluated by a few simple instruments to determine if the unit is performing as designed. Mea-

TABLE 4.11 Instruments Used for Incinerator Troubleshooting.

Measuring Device	What it Does	Purpose
Amp Probe	Measures motor current/ amperage	Indicates if a fan is handling the proper amount of gas
Manometer	Reads static pressure	Determines if sufficient negative pressure exists in the incinerator
System Thermometer	Measures gas temperature	Relates to combustion efficiency detection
Fyrite Kit or Orsat	Checks gas composition (oxygen and carbon dioxide)	Relates to combustion efficiency and excess air detection

surements of temperature and gas analyses indicate if the unit is operating properly, static pressure measurements indicate if there is enough draft in the unit, and fan speed and motor current indicate if the unit is supplying enough air or properly removing the combustion gases. Table 4.11 is a listing of some of the basic troubleshooting instruments.

In addition to these instruments, you can use a static pressure survey kit that allows you to troubleshoot an air system. This kit will determine the following:

- resistance in undersized ducts
- resistance in sharp turning elbows
- resistance across dry and wet collectors (also referred to as the pressure drop)
- static pressure of fans
- blockage of any sort in duct or collectors
- fugitive system problems
- fan horsepower

Readings obtained in the survey should be checked against manufacturer's specifications and any adjustments should be made in accordance with manufacturer's instructions.

4.3 SUMMARY

Chapter 3 notes that waste material can be successfully treated in an environmentally acceptable manner in a properly designed and operated incineration system. Even the best incinerator will fail to perform if maintained and operated improperly. Historically, too many hospital incinerators have not been operated in the proper manner. Operators must be adequately trained in the principles and procedures of incineration. The incinerator should be maintained to provide uniform and continuous operation with proper air, draft, feed, auxiliary fuel, and temperatures. Upsets should be avoided because they result in incomplete burnout and also in the formation of undesirable products of incomplete combustion (PICs). The feeding of infectious wastes during start-up and shutdown periods must be avoided to prevent the release of dangerous pathogens.

Incinerator operating data should be monitored and test burns conducted before burning infectious waste. The EPA recommends tests using a variety of *Bacillus subtillus* to see how many spores survive the burn under various operating conditions. Properly trained operators can optimize the system to ensure that infectious materials are properly destroyed.

Incinerators: Waste Heat Recovery, Retrofitting, Testing, and Regional Use

5.1 WASTE HEAT RECOVERY

WASTE Heat Recovery is a natural consideration when implementing an incineration system. The high-temperature gases typically generated offer an excellent source of energy with which to produce steam. Hospitals generally have sufficient demand to fully utilize steam generated through a waste heat recovery operation. Typical uses for steam within the hospital include laundry equipment, food preparation equipment, dishwashers, autoclaves, domestic hot water heating, and environmental heating.

For hospital applications, waste heat boilers of fire tube designs are most commonly used to effect the heat recovery process. A waste heat boiler is actually an ordinary fire tube boiler without a fuel burner. Exhaust gases are simply ducted from the incinerator to the boiler to supply the energy source to produce steam. Like a traditional fire tube boiler, waste heat recovery boilers are available in one-, two-, three-, and even four-pass designs.

Basic operating procedures are essentially the same for a waste heat boiler as for a traditional fire tube boiler. Proper feed water conditions must be maintained through chemical treatment.

There is one major concern, however, when operating a waste heat boiler with an incinerator: exhaust gas particulate content. Particulate, or fly ash, is a residue of the solid waste incineration process, and its presence simply means that a waste heat boiler must utilize a "dirtier" flue gas than that used in a fuel-fired boiler. The primary effect of using a "dirty" flue gas is an increased fouling of the boiler tubes that hinders the heat transfer process and thus reduces the boiler efficiency. To alleviate this problem, soot blowers should be installed.

Other areas that may require periodic cleaning due to particulate

101

buildup include the exhaust gas intake and the induced draft fan blades. Fouling of fan blades may decrease fan efficiency and thus increase the power required to maintain a proper draft on the system.

An excessive particulate concentration in the flue gas may indicate poor incineration performance. Proper incinerator operation is therefore vitally important in maintaining an efficient heat recovery process.

Accessories and auxiliary systems included with a waste heat recovery boiler will depend on the equipment available in the existing boiler plant. Existing feed water, chemical treatment, and blowdown systems may be used if appropriately sized to accommodate an additional boiler. Proximity to the existing main steam lines and boiler plant should be considered when sizing a waste-to-energy system.

For certain applications, it may be advantageous to install a multifuel-fired boiler. A multifuel-fired boiler offers the flexibility of operating in three modes: (1) waste heat only, (2) natural gas (or other fuel) only, and (3) waste heat and a second fuel together to achieve the full-rated capacity of the boiler. A significant advantage to this system is in the elimination of cycling between a waste heat boiler and a separate traditional fuel-fired boiler. In some cases, several older existing boilers may be replaced by a new, higher efficiency, multifuel-fired boiler to supply the hospital's base steam load.

5.1.1 OPERATION AND MAINTENANCE

Like all other devices, the waste heat boiler must be properly operated and maintained. These procedures are summarized in Table 5.1.

If not kept clean, the boiler tank heat transfer can be seriously degraded. The effect of soot on boiler fouling is shown in Table 5.2.

For reliable service, spare parts must be available. A suggested spare parts inventory is given in Table 5.3.

5.2 RETROFITTING

Many states including Florida, California, New York, New Jersey, Pennsylvania, and Indiana are considering or have already passed legisla-tion/regulations relative to the handling, transport, and disposal of infec-tious or biomedical wastes. These regulations include incinerator perfor-mance requirements such as those presented in section 3.2.4 (see Table 5.4) that address safety, residue burnout, secondary combustion chamber design, temperature and residence time, and also emissions limitations (i.e., HCl and particulates that will be presented in section 5.2.4).

TABLE 5.1 Waste Heat Boilers Operating and Maintenance Procedures.

Description	Frequency	Comments
Operate soot blowers (if manual)	Daily	Excessive buildup may require more frequent operation.
Check flue gas temperature	Daily	A temperature increase may be an indication of poor heat transfer. Boiler tubes may require more frequent cleaning.
Check flue gas pressure	Daily	An increase in pressure drop across the boiler may indicate fouling of the boiler tubes.
Check steam pressure	Daily	A decrease in steam pressure may indicate overloading of boiler.
Check burner (for multifuel-fired boiler)	Daily	Periodic cleaning may be necessary to maintain optimum burner performance.
Check blowdown	Daily	Excessive blowdown may result in significant heat loss and thus reduce boiler efficiency.
Check blowers	Weekly	Excessive fouling of fan blades may reduce fan efficiency and increase energy consumption.
Check gas inlet to boiler	Weekly	Excessive fouling of gas inlet may result in decrease of gas pressure.
Check dampers	Weekly	Excessive fouling may adversely affect the desired draft on the system.
Check water treatment procedures	Weekly	Insufficient treatment may result in scale buildup and/or corrosion.
Check valves	Monthly	Valve stems or packing may leak and lubrication may be necessary. Clean and recondition as necessary.
Check motors	Monthly	Clean and recondition as necessary.
Check pumps	Monthly	Clean and recondition as necessary.
Check electrical systems	Monthly	Clean terminals and replace any defective parts.

TABLE 5.2 Effect of Fouling on Boiler Efficiency.

Inches of Soot	Loss of Efficiency
1/32	9.5%
1/16	26 %
1/8	45 %
3/16	69 %

TABLE 5.3 Recommended Spare Parts List for Maintenance of Boiler.

Description	Quantity Required
Water Column Gage Glass	2
Gage Glass Seal	4
Gage Glass Washer	4
Handhole Gasket	4
Clean-Out Plug Gasket	1
Manway Gasket	1
Front Door Gasket and Installation Kit	1
Rear Door Gasket and Installation Kit	1
Sightglass for Rear Observation Port	2
Gasket for Rear Observation Port Sightglass	4
Touch-Up Paint, Aerosol Can	NA
Anti-Seize, Aerosol Can	1
Flue Brush	1
Low Water Cutoff Replacement Head	1
Operating Control	1
Limit Control	1
Firing Rate Control	1
Auxiliary Low Water Cutoff Relay	1
Flame Safeguard Programmer	1
Flame Safeguard Amplifier	1
Flame Safeguard Scanner	1
Ignition Electrode	2
Control Circuit Fuse	6
Air Flow Switch	1
Blower Wheel	1
Blower Motor	1
Modulator Motor	1
Indicating Lamp Replacement Bulbs/Lamp	1

TABLE 5.4 Infectious Waste Incineration Combustion Criteria.

Paremeter	Design/Performance Criteria
Burnout*	≥95%
Combustion Efficiency*	≥95%
Primary Chamber Temperature	≥1,500°F
Secondary Chamber Temperature	≥1,800°F
Secondary Chamber Gas Retention Time	1.0 to 2.0 Seconds

*See Section 3.2.4.

5.2.1 WHY RETROFIT

The major reason to retrofit an incinerator is to meet new regulations. Most of these regulations have a 6–12 month grace period before an existing incinerator is required to meet them or be shut down. An exception to this practice would be through the issuance of a Consent Order, which is a legal document issued by the regulatory agency, allowing a *scheduled delay* in completing the modification and installation of new equipment.

Some of the advantages of retrofitting are as follows:

- energy recovery (installation of a waste heat boiler)
- increased longevity of the existing system
- decreased liability (better destruction of waste)
- decreased environmental impact (reduction of emissions)

The major disadvantage of retrofitting is the cost.

5.2.2 SYSTEMATIC APPROACH

The first and perhaps most important step in the retrofitting of a hospital incinerator is to *evaluate* the condition of the existing system. New regulatory requirements must be met along with other goals that the hospital may want to achieve that may include increased incinerator capacity, energy recovery, and operator safety.

The next is to estimate the cost of retrofitting as compared to the installation of a new unit (see Figure 5.1). Usually, if the cost of the retrofit exceeds 60 percent of the cost of a new unit, it is advisable to replace the existing incinerator with a new one.

Once retrofitting is completed, it will be necessary to test the system and obtain a new air permit for operation. If an air pollution control system is added or there is *substantial* modification to the incinerator, a new air pollution construction permit may also be required prior to retrofit construction.

5.2.3 ALTERNATIVES

Various retrofitting alternatives designed to enhance the performance of the existing system are available as shown in Figure 5.2. The one common change in most states is to increase the waste *retention time* in the secondary chamber from 0.25–0.50 seconds up to 1–2 seconds, along with raising *temperatures* from 1,600–1,800°F. Other optional requirements will vary from state to state.

Another area that regulators consider important involves the residue quality of the ash/noncombustibles being removed from the primary com-

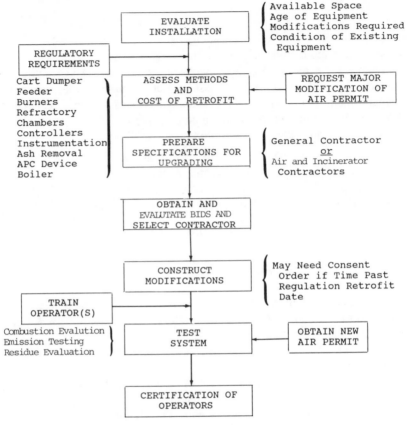

Figure 5.1 Systematic approach to the retrofit of an infectious waste incineration system including emission control and ash handling systems.

bustion chamber because incinerators may be required to achieve 95–99 percent burnout. Many of the other options available for retrofitting are illustrated in Figure 5.3, along with the type of improvement that may be expected from the upgrading of the facility.

5.2.4 MEETING EMISSION REQUIREMENTS

The new air pollution emission requirements are very restrictive and include regulations for particulates, acid gases, opacity, and other components as noted in Table 5.5.

These more restrictive requirements may require the addition of a wet or dry scrubber system to control particulates and acid gases. Normally, a

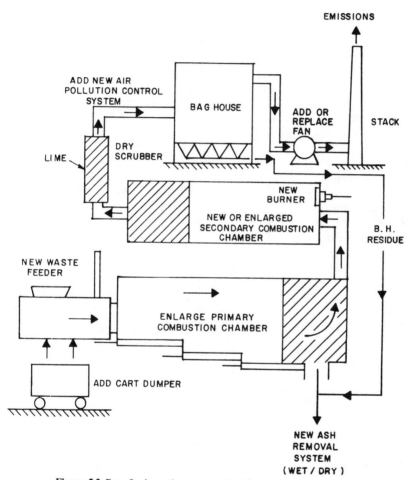

Figure 5.2 Retrofit alternatives to upgrade infectious waste incinerators.

RETROFIT ITEM	TYPE OF IMPROVEMENT EXPECTED								
	SAFETY	COMBUSTION EFFICIENCY (PRIMARY)	VOC DESTRUCTION (SECONDARY)	RESIDUE BURNOUT	REDUCE PARTICULATE EMISSIONS	REDUCE HCl EMISSIONS	ASH REMOVAL	COMBUSTION CONTROL	ENERGY RECOVERY
CART DUMPER	★								
RAM FEEDER	★	★							
LONGER PRIMARY			★	★					
BIGGER BURNER			★					★	
LONGER SECONDARY			★		★			★	
ASH CONVEYOR	★			★					
AIR MODULATION		★	★	★	★			★	
COMPUTER CONTROL		★	★	★	★		★	★	
MONITORING DEV. (CO,O_2,HCl, Opac.)	★	★	★	★	★			★	
VENTURI SCRUBBER					★				
PACKED TOWER						★			
LARGER/NEW FAN		★	★	★	★			★	
WASTE HEAT BOILER									★

Figure 5.3 Retrofit improvements for infectious waste incinerators.

TABLE 5.5 Range of Emission Limits for Hospital Incinerators.

Pollutant	Emission Range
Particulate	0.1–0.015 gr/scf @ 7% O_2[1]
Hydrochloric Acid (HCl)	30–50 ppmv[2]
	90% Removed
	51 lb/h
Opacity	5–40%
Carbon Monoxide (CO)	50–100 ppmv
Sulfur Dioxide (SO_2)	30–50 ppmv

[1] gr/scf @ 7% O_2 = grains/standard cubic foot corrected to 7 percent oxygen
[2] ppmv = parts per million by volume

controlled-air incinerator produces relatively low gaseous emissions and particulates. In a regional facility where either a rotary kiln or controlled-air unit may be used, however, a particulate control device will be required to meet many state regulatory requirements. In addition, due to a relatively high waste content of chlorinated plastics, acid gas emissions will also need to be controlled with an absorber.

In order to meet the new requirements, complicated control devices may be required that will increase costs considerably and will require rather sophisticated operation. A facility retrofitting or installing an incinerator at this time should consider the installation of air pollution control equipment now or allow space for adding this equipment as it becomes a requirement in the future.

5.2.5 RETROFIT COSTS

The cost of retrofitting an incinerator system is dependent upon the capital cost of the required equipment and on the amount of labor necessary for installation. The labor costs are based upon a local contractor or a manufacturer's service representative's rates and usually includes daily and overtime rates, layover time, and transportation/travel time.

Typical capital costs for retrofit items are included in Table 5.6; the manpower requirements for installation are tabulated in Table 5.7; and typical service representative charges are listed in Table 5.8.

The cost to retrofit air pollution control equipment was given in Table 5.6 and the cost of new incinerators was presented in Figure 3.7. Using the information from these two items, a typical example of how to cost a retrofit system is provided.

Example Problem

Upgrade a five-year-old ECP, batch type, 500 lb/h controlled-air incinerator to meet the new Indiana regulations.

TABLE 5.6 Retrofit of Hospital (Infectious Waste) Incinerators Capital Costs (1988 Dollars).

Added Equipment	Size (lb/h)		
	600	800	1000
Feed System			
—Add Ram Feed	20,000	20,000	21,000
—Add Cart Dumper	12,000	15,000	18,000
Primary Combustion Chamber			
Correct Leaks			
—Around Feeder	2,000	2,000	2,000
—Guillotine Damper	2,000	2,000	2,000
Refractory			
—Champber-Kaocrete 28LI	7,000	7,500	8,000
—Hearth-Brick	2,000	2,500	3,000
Add Burner	4,500	4,500	5,000
Extended Chamber for Burnout	10,000	12,000	14,000
Ash Removal System			
—Add Wet System	24,000	24,000	30,000
—Add Dry System	30,000	35,000	40,000
—Add Hood to Existing Dry System			
Secondary Combustion Chamber			
Refractory			
—Chamber	9,000	9,500	10,000
—Flameport	200	200	200
—Add Burner (High Capacity)			
(Up to 1800°F)			
Packaged Block Type	4,500	4,500	5,000
Enlarge S.C.C.			
(For Retention Time) (i.e., 2 s)	$250/ft^3	$250/ft^3	$250/ft^3
Waste Heat Boiler			
—Add New Boiler	47,000	47,000	82,000
—Add Soot Blowers	12,000	12,000	15,000
Air Pollution Control System			
—Venturi Packed Tower—Complete	180,000	210,000	230,000
—Dry/Dry Scrubber—Non-RCRA	230,000	270,000	300,000
Fan			
—Add New Fan (Larger Capacity) with Silencer	7,500	9,000	10,000
Controls			
—Variable Air Control		20,000	
—Process Controller		28,000 (+ site work)	

TABLE 5.6 (Continued).

Added Equipment	Size (lb/h)		
	600	800	1000
Monitoring Devices			
Combustion			
—O_2	13,000	13,000	13,000
—CO_2	15,000	15,000	15,000
—CO	16,000	16,000	16,000
(no recorders)			
Environmental			
—Opacity	29,000	29,000	29,000
Testing			
—Thermocouples—Type R	350	350	350
—Pressure Gages	350	350	350

Note: Does not include field service. Please refer to attached schedule of charges.

TABLE 5.7 Manpower Requirements for Retrofit of Hospital (Infectious Waste) Incinerators.[1]

Added Equipment	Days	Personnel
Feed System		
—Add Ram Feed	4–5	2 (1 + helper) + Crane ($1000)
—Add Cart Dumper	1	2 (1 + helper)
Primary Combustion Chamber		
Correct Leaks		
—Around Feeder	1	1
—Guillotine Damper	1	1
Refractory		
(Remove and replace whole chamber)		
—Chamber	5	3
—Hearth	5	3
Add Burner		
Extend Chamber for Burnout (Add 4 Feet)	10	4
Ash Removal System		
—Add Wet System	10	4
—Add Dry System	10	4
—Add Hood to Existing Dry System	No Problem	

(continued)

TABLE 5.7 (Continued).

Added Equipment	Days	Personnel
Secondary Combustion Chamber		
Refractory		
—Chamber	5	3
—Flameport	1	1
—Add Burner (High Capacity)	3	2
(Up to 1800°F)		
Enlarge S.C.C.		
(For Retention Time) (i.e., 2 s)	10	4
Waste Heat Boiler		
—Add New Boiler	5	3
		(Crane $2,000)
—Add Soot Blowers	1	1
Air Pollution Control System		
—Venturi Packed Tower	10	2
—Dry/Dry Scrubber	20	2
Fan		
—Add New Fan (Larger Capacity)	1	1
Controls		
—Variable Air Control	2	1
—Process Controller	4–7	2
Monitoring Devices		
Combustion		
—O_2	1	1
—CO_2	1	1
—CO	1	1
Environmental		
—Opacity	1	1
Testing		
—Thermocouples	2	1
—Pressure Gages	2	1

[1]600–1,000 lb/h capacity.

TABLE 5.8 Typical Net Charges for Service Representatives.

The net charges for a service representative are determined in accordance with the following schedule: meals, lodging, travel, expenses, miscellaneous expenses and transportation are charged as incurred plus a 15 percent carrying charge.

Working 8-hour day (Monday thru Friday)	$550 per day
Overtime hours in excess of 8 hours per day	$103 per hour
Saturdays	$103 per hour
Sundays and Holidays	$140 per hour

Layover Time—No Work Performed

Monday thru Friday	$550 per day
Holidays, Saturdays, and Sundays	$550 per day
Meals and Lodging	As Incurred, plus 15% carry-ing charge

Transportation and Travel Time

Transportation	As Incurred, plus 15% carry-ing charge
Travel Time—Monday thru Friday	$50 per day
Saturdays and Sundays	$103 per hour
Holidays	$137 per hour
Minimum Charge for Fraction of the Day	$550 per day

Areas That Would Require Upgrading:

- add a cart dumper
- add a ram feeder
- add an ash removal system
- enlarge the secondary combustion chamber (go from 0.5 to 1 s retention time)
- add a new secondary burner

The results are summarized in Table 5.9. The conclusion is that the cost of the upgrade is $138,700 and the cost of a new unit would be approximately $250,000. The upgraded figure represents 56 percent of the cost of a new unit; therefore, it would be better to replace the unit.

5.3 SOURCE TESTING

This section is not intended to be a detailed discussion on incineration source-testing procedures because source testing is a very complex, exact

TABLE 5.9 Summary of Estimated Cost of Upgrading.

Item to Upgrade	Capital Cost $	Additional Labor Costs					Expenses ($)	Total Cost ($)
		Days	Personnel	Total MDs	Cost ($)			
Cart Dumper	12,000	1	1	1	550		50	12,600
Ram Feeder	20,000	5	2	10	5,500		500	26,000
Ash Removal System	24,000[a]	10	4	40	22,000		2,000	48,000
Enlarge Secondary Combustion Chamber	20,000[b]	10	4	40	22,000		2,000	44,000
New Secondary Burner	4,500	3	2	6	3,300		300	8,100
Total	80,500	29	13	97	53,350		4,850[c]	138,700

[a]Wet System
[b]Add 10 feet, 3.2' diameter (For a 0.5 s retention time, the chamber was 10 ft long and its volume was 80 ft³).
[c]Probably Low

process that should be left to trained specialists. However, to evaluate and eventually control either potential or existing air pollution problems, the types and amounts of emissions from a source or group of sources must be shown. There are seven primary reasons for determining source emission level data.

The first reason is to determine whether or not a particular source is in compliance with proposed or existing emission regulations set forth by governmental agencies. For example, to implement air pollution control strategies and to meet ambient air quality standards, the 1970 Clean Air Act allows the Environmental Protection Agency (EPA) Administrator to require performance emission tests and written reports. Furthermore, individual states also have the authority to require source tests on any stationary source.

A second reason is to incorporate a registration system into the regulatory process. The results of a source test are often used to determine the issuance, denial, or revocation of any permit to operate equipment that is a potential or actual source of contaminant emissions.

Third, source tests are essential to determine the efficiency of control equipment installed to reduce pollutant emissions. An industry or governmental agency may require such a performance test prior to the final acceptance of a newly installed control device. Such a test usually involves either a comparison of tests conducted before and after installing the control equipment or testing of the effluent entering and discharged from the control equipment.

Fourth, source-test data are invaluable in selecting or designing appropriate control equipment. Such data are frequently helpful in modifying either the basic process or the equipment involved.

Fifth, accumulated data from source-sampling tests and analyses are useful in identifying predominant sources of specific contaminants. This is often referred to as an "emission inventory." Such information often leads to the recognition of the need for new or revised control regulations that establish or tighten emission limitations on these sources.

Sixth, research and development may be very much affected by source-test data, particularly concerning the development and implementation of new or modified processes that may be potential emission sources.

Finally, the seventh reason is similar to the sixth in that it involves loss control and process control. In controlling losses from a given process, source sampling frequently identifies excessive losses of product or raw materials that are given off as emissions. Periodic source tests are often conducted to determine if a given process is operating efficiently. Malfunctions can sometimes be diagnosed from these tests. In some cases, such tests are an economic necessity since inefficient operations over a length of time result in lost resource materials and thus, lost profits.

5.3.1 BASIC REQUIREMENTS OF SOURCE TESTING

Regardless of the eventual application, the immediate objective in source testing is obtaining reliable data on the effluent composition and rate of emission to the atmosphere. The following requirements are basic to any source test:

(1) The gas stream being sampled must be representative of either the total or a known portion of the source emissions.
(2) Collected samples must be representative of the gas stream being sampled.
(3) The gas sample volume must be measured to allow calculation of concentrations in the sampled gas stream.
(4) The gas flow rate must be determined to allow calculation of emission rates.
(5) Physical measurements must be made of the temperature, pressure, moisture content, etc., of the sample and the stack gases so that the gas law computations can be performed.

5.3.2 GENERAL PROCEDURES

From initial planning to final report, a source-test procedure consists of a number of steps, the scope of each depending upon the complexity of the test program. Normally, these steps are performed in the following order:

(1) Establishing the requirements for the source test
(2) Inspecting the source for physical test requirements
(3) Selecting the test procedures
(4) Scheduling the tests
(5) Measuring the gas velocity and flow rate
(6) Collecting the samples
(7) Processing and analyzing the samples
(8) Making calculations from field and laboratory data
(9) Preparing the test report

Planning a source test requires that the objective(s) be defined, i.e., is the test to determine compliance with regulations, check the performance of an existing control device, establish the need for a control device, etc. Such planning includes estimating the types and amounts of pollutant emissions (by use of emission factors or material balance), the flow rates and the problems that may be encountered, as well as determining the particular pollutant to be sampled.

A physical inspection of the source is used to establish the location(s) for sampling ports, as well as requirements for platforms, scaffolding, accessibility, availability of electrical power, operating schedules, etc. Preliminary determinations of temperature, velocity, pressure, and moisture content of the gas streams should also be made at this time. Personnel safety and minimum exposure to adverse weather conditions must also be considered.

The test procedures and equipment employed must be suitable to the particular test, taking into account such factors as the test objectives, governmental control requirements, suitability of the data, usefulness of the data in potential legal actions, and any other applicable considerations. Furthermore, the versatility, efficiency, usability, and accuracy of the test equipment itself must be evaluated.

When scheduling source tests, allowances must be made for the contracting of personnel and equipment, the development of special test methods, the coordination with plant management personnel, and the operation of the facility (must be under conditions specified for the test). For example, in cyclical (or other nonuniform) operations, the sampling times must be determined prior to actual sampling, and they may be established so as to take advantage of the varying conditions. To allow for study, preparation, flow measurement, analyses, calculations, and report preparation, four to six off-stack man hours must be allowed for each man hour of sample collection. Generally, a full working day is needed for a two- or three-man crew to collect two or three particulate samples.

For computing both concentrations and mass emission rates, the rate of gas flow and flow conditions must be accurately measured. In order to establish accurate gas flow parameters, it is necessary to make accurate measurements of velocity, temperature, static pressure, gas composition and density, and cross-sectional area. Such flow measurements are made just prior to actual sample collection.

In collecting a sample, a known volume of gas is withdrawn from the stack or duct through a sampling train. The amount of gas withdrawn, the equivalent volume at source conditions, and the amount of collected materials must all be measured.

In normal practice, the collected sample is transported to a laboratory for analysis. Analysis should be accurately accomplished in accordance with specified procedures. Analytical methods should always be as accurate and as simple as possible. Since gaseous and particulate analytical methods are well described in other texts, this book shall not attempt to duplicate their description.

Following sample collection and analysis, appropriate calculations are used to determine concentrations and emission rates for particulate and gaseous emissions. Such calculations are based on a knowledge of the gas flow rate and conditions, the equivalent gas volume taken as a sample, and the amount of material collected.

At the conclusion of the test study, a report is prepared to document the procedures used, the purpose of the test, and the findings. Normally the report consists of seven sections: (1) the test purpose; (2) a process description including the operating parameters and flow diagram; (3) pertinent facts, including date, time location, plant, and test personnel; (4) a description of the sampling and analytical methods and the calculations, including sketches of the sampling train and the analytical apparatus; (5) raw and final data from the test; (6) the results in terms of significant trends, predicted or theoretical results, and sampling anomalies; and (7) the conclusions and recommendations based on the data evaluation and limitations. A result summary, such as the one shown in Table 5.10, should be included.

Source testing is a complex and often difficult task. Some measurements (e.g., velocity and temperature) must be taken inside of the stack or duct, while most other measurements regarding the actual composition of the stack gas are taken externally. Both types of measurements are affected by the process conditions.

5.3.3 PROCESS CONDITIONS AND EMISSION FACTORS

There are wide variations in process conditions in most operations, resulting in differing characteristics and quantities of gaseous emissions.

TABLE 5.10 Typical Stack Sampling Results.
Controlled-Air Incinerator Burning Infectious (Hospital) Wastes—
Summary of Results: Particulate, HCl Acid, and CO Sampling.

Run Number	1	2	3
Date	08/09/88	08/09/88	08/09/88
% Isokinetic	100.46	103.01	104.04
Volume of Gas Sampled,[1] scf (Dry)	38.45	38.88	39.68
Stack Gas Flow Rate,[1] scfm (Dry)	2808.0	2722.2	2737.6
Stack Gas Flow Rate, acfm	7173.89	7056.3	7167.1
Particulate:			
Catch, mg	52.32	60.01	70.31
Concentration, grains/scf = Dry	0.0229	0.0264	0.0304
Concentration, grains/scf = Dry @ 12% CO_2	0.0557	0.0634	0.0719
Emission Rate, lb/h	0.550	0.615	0.714
HCl Acid:			
Catch, mg	686.7	944.8	1095.6
Concentration,[1] grains/scf (Dry)	0.3000	0.4152	0.4740
Emission Rate, lb/h	7.219	9.687	11.121
Carbon Monoxide:			
Concentration, ppm (dry basis)	16	4	6

[1]At 68°F, 29.92 in Hg.

Where more than one source exhausts to the same stack or duct, additional fluctuations may occur. Since sampling procedures require considerable lengths of time, the sampling method and/or conditions must frequently be changed to account for these variations in the process conditions.

A prerequisite of source testing is a knowledge of the conditions (i.e., gas velocity, temperature, and pressure) inside the stack. The equipment used to conduct these measurements must be capable of withstanding a highly corrosive environment. Furthermore, poor mixing conditions within the stack or duct often necessitate taking these measurements at many points, which tends to greatly lengthen the time required for conducting a source test.

The sampling team must be properly prepared before going into the field by having familiarized themselves with the unit operation or process that they intend to check. The primary purpose of source testing is to verify what is already known about the source, not to determine things not already known. One means of estimating the contents of an effluent gas is through the use of emission factors and handbook data. For example, suppose it is necessary to test a 250 ton/day municipal incinerator. It is necessary to estimate the moisture content of the stack gases; the stack gas temperature; the range of emissions expected, including grain loading and mass emission rate; and the amount of excess air.

From published reference sources that include emission factors, it would be possible to determine the following:

(1) The moisture content of the stack gases from the incinerator furnace would range between 20 and 30 percent.
(2) The excess air would range from 200 to 300 percent.
(3) The average stack temperature, depending upon moisture content and excess air, would range between 600 and 1600°F.
(4) The amount of stack gas could be as high as
$$250 \text{ t/d} \times 400 \text{ cfm/t} = 100,000 \text{ acfm}$$
(5) By taking the emission factor of 30 lb/t for uncontrolled multiple-chamber municipal incinerators, the mass emission rate equals
$$250 \text{ t/d} \times 30 \text{ lb/h} \times 1 \text{ d/24h} = 313 \text{ lb/h}$$
(6) The concentration would then equal
$$313 \text{ lb/h} \times 7000 \text{ gr/lb} \times 1 \text{ h/60 min} \times \frac{1}{100,000 \text{ acfm}} = 0.365 \text{ gr/acf}$$

5.3.4 SAMPLING THEORY

Obviously, the total gas stream of a stack or duct cannot be put through the sampling device. Therefore, a part of the gas must be sampled and analyzed as shown in Figure 5.4. After determining the pollutant mass con-

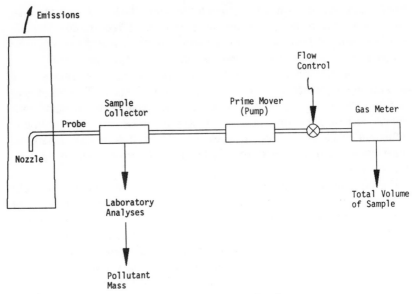

Figure 5.4 Simplified source sampling diagram.

centration and the gas volume flow rate of the stack or duct, the total pollutant mass emission rate can be calculated. To determine this rate, a representative sample must be obtained, efficiently collected and preserved, and then properly analyzed. Each of these operations entails numerous steps, any of which provides considerable opportunity for the introduction of errors.

For accurate source sampling, the collected sample should be *representative* of the actual stack gas; it should have the same characteristics, in the same relationship, as the parent gas from which it was taken. A sample containing either more or less pollutant than the stack gas is *nonrepresentative* or *biased*. For widely fluctuating stack conditions, proportional or isokinetic sampling must be used. In the field, considerable effort is directed toward obtaining a truly representative sample.

To avoid sample loss due to absorption, condensation, chemical reactions, settling, impingement, or other means, the sampling equipment should be located as near as possible to the actual sampling point. Furthermore, the efficiency of the collection device must be known and the total amount of collected gas must be determined. Only then can the concentrations and emission rates be accurately calculated.

Once removed from the stack, the sample must be transported without any changes. The design of the sampling equipment (e.g., nozzle, probe, etc.) must preclude physical or chemical changes in the sample during collection and extreme care must be exercised to preserve the sample after collection as well. Improper handling of the collected sample can easily void all precautions taken during the actual sampling process.

The performance of the analytical process requires an adequate amount of sample, and size-of-sample considerations often dictate how the test will be conducted. To avoid problems of reagent and/or sample deterioration, analysis should be taken as soon as possible after collection and standard procedures should always be followed.

Most existing plants were not designed for source testing, so finding a suitable location is frequently a problem. It is often difficult to find an accessible and safe area to locate the sampling ports, especially one that allows for the manipulation of the necessary equipment. In addition, the location should be removed from obstructions in the stack or duct that would disturb the gas flow. While sampling tests can still be performed under such circumstances, there is usually a need for a greater number of samples in order to be representative. The task is, as a result, considerably more difficult and time-consuming.

5.3.5 SAFETY CONSIDERATIONS

For a variety of reasons, source sampling can be a hazardous task. Many sources contain toxic constituents and the only available sampling locations may be well above the ground, situated on temporary scaffolding. Since the sampling equipment requires electrical power, there is danger of electrical shorts, especially during inclement weather. Personnel safety should always be of primary importance, and the test procedure and environment must always comply with state and federal regulations. (The Federal 1970 Occupational Safety and Health Act is pertinent to all such cases.)

5.3.6 PARTICULATE SAMPLING

Particulate sampling is often more complicated than gas sampling. Depending on the reason for sampling, the variety and extent of components used in the sampling train will vary. For example, if the chemical and physical characteristics of the aerosols are to be measured, a multicomponent train, or even multiple sampling trains, may be required. On the other hand, if mass loading alone is being measured, a lesser number of components will be needed.

With particulate sampling, unlike gas sampling, more attention needs to be focused on the sampling rate because representative sampling can be obtained only if the velocity of the stack gas stream entering the probe nozzle is the same as the velocity of the stream passing the nozzle. If the sampling velocity is too high (super-isokinetic sampling), there will be a smaller concentration of particles collected (because the inertia of the larger particles prevents them from following the stream lines into the nozzle). Alternatively, in sub-isokinetic sampling, where the sampling velocity is below that of the flowing gas stream, the gas samples would contain a higher-than-actual particulate concentration (because heavier aerosol particles will enter the nozzle but light particles will be diverted). Figure 5.5 illustrates isokinetic, super-isokinetic and sub-isokinetic flow.

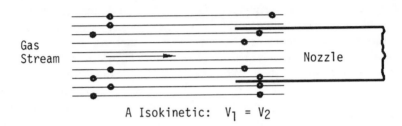

A Isokinetic: $V_1 = V_2$

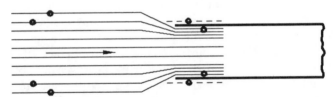

B Super-Isokinetic: V_1 larger than V_2

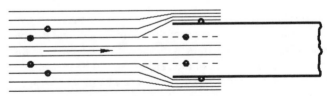

C Sub-Isokinetic: V_1 less than V_2

KEY:
V_1 = GAS STREAM LOCAL VELOCITY
V_2 = SAMPLE NOZZLE VELOCITY

Figure 5.5 Particle sampling and collection velocity.

It has been found that inertia effects become more significant when particle diameters exceed about 3 microns; therefore, if a reasonable proportion of the particles exceed this size, isokinetic sampling is necessary.

The Environmental Protection Agency requires that the sampling conditions must be within 10 percent isokinetic (nozzle velocity/stack velocity) or the samples are to be rejected and the sampling repeated. Even samples within this range, they say, should be corrected by means of a complicated expression. Naturally, such correction factors are based on the assumption of a *normal* particle size distribution. If a source contains an unusual distribution, correction factors must be avoided. In many cases, isokinetic sampling (with or without correction factors) is used without particle size data, since isokinetic conditions are needed to obtain valid samples for particle size distribution evaluations.

The probe nozzle is selected, after accounting for changes in temperature, pressure, and moisture content (from condensation) in the train, so that the pump can maintain isokinetic velocity. For measurements at a single point, pump maintenance may not be difficult, but for multipoint sampling (which is most common) the mathematical and physical manipulations are often troublesome.

5.3.7 SYSTEM MONITORING

In addition to source testing, system parameters should be monitored to validate unit operation and are summarized in Table 5.11. The device locations are shown in Figure 5.6.

In addition to the control of particulates, opacity, and odors, recent air emission control regulations, as proposed and adopted by state agencies, have been directed toward the following:

(1) More stringent control of particulates

(2) Control of acid gases, especially hydrochloric acid (HCl)

(3) Control of carbon monoxide (CO).

The more stringent control of particulates can be attributed to the availability of improved control technology, while the control of acid gases has been prompted by the amount of chlorinated plastics contained in hospital waste. An EPA study [1] shows that hospital waste may contain between 20 to 30 percent plastics made up of primarily polyethylene, polypropylene, and polyvinyl chloride (PVC) with PVC being approximately 45 percent chlorine.

This large quantity of chlorine may cause combustion products that include HCl and toxic organic compounds. EPA emission data, as presented in the study, shows HCl concentrations ranging from 40 to 2,095 ppmv for

TABLE 5.11 **Incinerator System Monitors (Type and Location).**

Location	Parameter	Type Sensor	Position	Comments
Primary Combustion Chamber	Temperature	Thermocouple	Flame Port	Type R Thermocouple Range: 0 to 3000°F
Secondary Combustion Chamber	Temperature	Thermocouple	In Breeching at End of Chamber	Type R Thermocouple Range: 0 to 3000°F
	Oxygen	Paramagnetic	At Exit of Chamber	Needs to be Calibrated (Manually)
Waste Heat Boiler	Temperature	Thermocouple	Inlet and Outlet	Type R Thermocouple Range: 0 to 3000°F
	Pressure	Pressure Gauge	Inlet & Outlet	Type K Thermocouple Range: 0 to 2000°F
	Feed Water	Thermocouple	Inlet	Type K Thermocouple Range: 0 to 2000°F
Air Pollution Control System	Pressure Drop	Manometer	Refer to narration of Chapter 5	• Across Baghouse • Across Packed Tower • Across Mist Eliminator
	Water Flow	Orifice	Recirculation Pump Outlet	
Stack	Opacity	Transmissometer	Laminar Flow Zone	Needs to be Calibrated (Manually)
Fan	AMPS	AMP Probe	Fan Motor	Done Manually
	RPM	Tachometer	Fan Shaft	Done Manually

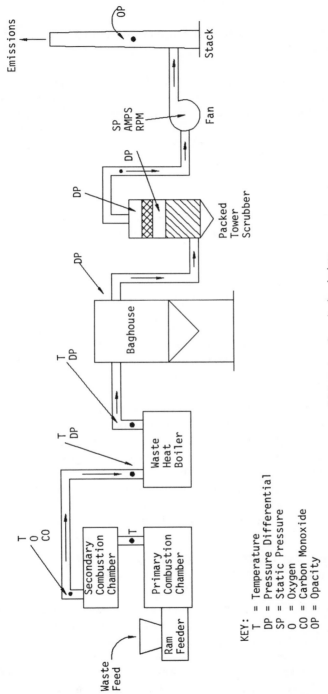

Figure 5.6 Location of monitoring devices.

KEY: T = Temperature
DP = Pressure Differential
SP = Static Pressure
O = Oxygen
CO = Carbon Monoxide
OP = Opacity

uncontrolled hospitals, with many hospitals being in the range of 550 to 1,000 ppmv [1].

The control of carbon monoxide is used as an indicator of the control of other organic compound emissions. Use of carbon monoxide serving as an indicator is discussed by the ASME Research Committee on Industrial and Municipal Waste [2]. The minimization of carbon monoxide emissions indicates the maximization of combustion efficiency and also the minimization of other organic compound emissions.

5.3.8 FIELD INSPECTION REPORT

Appendix 2 contains an example of a field inspection report for an incineration facility. Use this form as a guide to construct one suited to your specific application.

5.4 OFF-SITE REGIONAL INCINERATION FACILITIES

In the past, infectious waste combustion regulations were directed toward the control of particulates, opacity, and odors, but recently, new performance standards and guidelines also include the control of principal organic hazardous compounds (POHCs) and the products of incomplete combustion (PICs). The new performance standards may include requirements for combustion efficiency, burnout, minimum temperatures and gas retention times in the primary and secondary combustion chambers. Some of the typical performance criteria and their range of values were presented in Table 5.4. These additional criteria may suggest a regional approach to the infectious waste combustion process.

See Table 3.3 for a summary of current existing and/or proposed hospital incinerator state regulations. These regulations present controlled emission levels that reflect concern for the pollutants previously discussed.

5.4.1 COMPLIANCE WITH CURRENT AND PROPOSED EMISSION REGULATIONS

Compliance with the proposed and/or existing emission regulations included in Table 3.3 requires the use of current state-of-the-art control technology that is needed when emission regulations for both particulate and acid gas emissions are extremely stringent. For example, the proposed New York regulations require that particulate emissions not exceed 0.015 gr/dscf and HCl emissions, 50 ppmv. A review of existing controlled emission levels for hospitals, as listed in the EPA *Hospital Waste Combustion*

Study [1], shows that only fabric filters (baghouses) have achieved the required level of particulate control while only packed towers have achieved the 50 ppmv level of HCl control. These findings present somewhat of a dilemma in meeting both requirements because no existing single air pollution control concept has demonstrated the aforementioned combined limits for hospital-type facilities.

A relatively new concept, the dry scrubber with baghouse, has been proposed as a solution to this dilemma. Unfortunately, this optimism was due to the success of these systems in controlling particulates and acid gases in large waste-to-energy facilities (2,000 tons/day). However, the dry scrubber/baghouse combination has not been successfully applied to 10 to 20 ton/day hospital incinerators.

Some possible current solutions that would allow hospital incinerators to meet both the particulate and HCl emissions limitations are (1) the use of a fabric filter for emission control and the elimination of chlorinated plastics from hospital incinerator waste or (2) the use of a fabric filter in combination with a packed tower or a wet scrubber.

Based on the above combustion and emission criteria, future infectious waste incinerator configurations may exhibit some of the following combustion design considerations:

(1) Higher operating temperatures in the primary combustion chamber (1,500 to 1,800°F) to ensure good burnout and maximize destruction of pathogenic organisms

(2) More oxygen availability in the primary combustion chamber to minimize the formation of PICs

(3) Higher operating temperatures in the secondary combustion chamber (1,800 to 2,000°F) with increased gas retention times (1.0 to 2.0 seconds) to ensure destruction of organic compounds and any pathogenic organisms.

(4) Addition of mixing devices and/or mixing enhancements in the secondary combustion chamber to increase the destruction efficiency of organic compounds.

Air pollution control systems to control particulate and acid gases will become more common in the use and design of infectious waste incinerators.

5.4.2 POTENTIAL LIABILITY

Operating incinerator facilities can increase the possibility for liability suits. The liabilities that can result from the disposal of hospital waste at an off-site infectious waste disposal facility are a direct outcome of the design and operation of the facility and can cause serious in-plant or community-related problems.

The potential impacts that can occur from this type of facility can result in the following:

- fire
- explosion
- surface water pollution
- ground water contamination
- odor
- noise
- air pollution
- transportation accidents

These impacts can occur at any time and that is why management resolve, operational procedures, good equipment, good operator training, and good operation and management are necessary to minimize these potential hazards.

The liabilities that may occur can be categorized into the following groups:

(1) Public Related
- can affect the company reputation
- may limit future expansion
(2) Company Related
- insurance
- increased maintenance costs
- increased operational costs
- closure problems (bonding)
(3) Regulatory Related
- enforcement action
- fines
- nonissuance or withdrawal of permits
(4) Law Related
- damage suits
- nuisance suits

5.4.3 SITING

Many hospitals have some type of on-site thermal treatment device to treat pathological and infectious wastes. The most common types of thermal devices are sterilizers (autoclaves) and incinerators. The majority of the larger hospitals utilize on-site incinerators to destroy most of their wastes and thus reduce the liabilities associated with off-site land disposal facilities.

The siting process for an infectious waste incinerator must be endured whether the proposed facility will serve a single hospital or a service area that would include a number of hospitals, laboratories, veterinary clinics, or other users.

A regional facility serving a defined geographical area may be more easily sited from engineering and cost considerations because of the availability of a number of potential sites. Siting a regional facility that is not at a hospital may, however, bring more public attention. For this reason, future regional incinerators may be located at the site of an existing hospital.

Some of the major points to consider in siting a regional incinerator are as follows:

- Try to blend the incinerator in with the decor of the hospital. (This usually means enclosing the unit within a building connected with the hospital.)
- Keep fugitive dust, odors, noise, and visible emissions to a minimum through proper design and operation.
- Provide a stack that is aesthetically pleasing, yet at the same time, provides good dispersion of stack gases. (Short stacks can cause particulate disposition problems, odors, or even acid fallout.)

Other siting considerations are presented in Table 5.12.

A regional infectious waste incineration facility has to be carefully located because of economic (waste haul distance and location of potential energy customers) and environmental impact considerations.

To minimize transportation costs, a regional facility must be located within a minimum haul distance from the source(s) of infectious waste. Due to increased public awareness and concern regarding the handling and transportation of infectious waste, special disposable containers may be needed. These containers (boxes with plastic liners) are usually transported in refrigerated vehicles and immediately burned at the facility or placed in a cold storage room for future incineration.

It is advantageous to consider a buffer zone around a regional incineration facility to reduce the possible impact of particulate fallout, odors, noise, or other aesthetics problems. All too often, the individual hospital or regional facility is located too close to a residential area.

A regional hospital waste incineration facility should be located, whenever possible, so that the facility:

- creates the least environmental impact
- can provide steam to a commercial establishment or a co-op laundry operated by several hospitals
- minimizes transportation distance from the hospitals being served

TABLE 5.12 Consideration in Siting a Regional Hospital Incinerator.

Consideration	Issue	If Properly Done	If Improperly Done
Design	Stack Height	Dispenses emissions effectively	Causes downwash and citizen complaints
	Minimize Waste Transport	Reduces cost and handling of waste	May expose infectious waste to public
	Location at hospital	Aesthetically pleasing	Community eyesore
	Proper Design and Permitting of Incinerator	Incinerator installed promptly Properly sized for the hospital	Incinerator will have ongoing capacity and ash disposal problems
Operation and Maintenance	Operator Training	Reduces operating costs and environmental impact	Causes malfunctions and community nuisance and awareness
	Start-Up Shutdown	Reduces smoke and emissions	Causes community nuisance
	Safety	Waste handled effectively	Could be a liability problem
Environmental	Noise	Little or no noise	Noise from fans, motors, dampers and pumps
	Odor	No odor	If operating temperature is too low, odors will ensue
	Ash Disposal	No fugitive emissions	Odors and fugitive emissions
Stack Emissions	Particulates	No settleable particulates in community	Fly ash settling in community
	Hydrochloric Acid	No materials damage	Could be a problem to auto finishes or other materials damage from acid fallout
	Smoke	Zero visible emissions	Constant eyesore
	Health-Related Emissions (Spores)	No emissions	Possible community impact

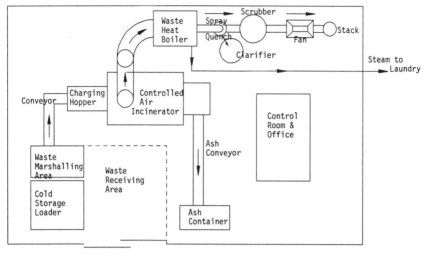

Figure 5.7 Typical hospital controlled-air incineration system.

5.4.4 OPERATION

The waste handling philosophy employed by regional facilities is to containerize the hospital wastes in heavy cardboard boxes (40 lb/box), double lined with plastic, and transport them by refrigerated van or truck to the regional facility. The disposal containers are either fed directly into the incinerator from the marshaling area (see Figure 5.7) or stored in a cold storage locker.

Consideration should be given to designing and permitting the facility as an infectious waste incinerator with the intent of re-permitting the system as a RCRA incinerator (RCRA B Permit) after it is up and running. In this way, the regional facility could eventually handle all of the hospital's infectious wastes and quantities of hazardous waste.

In the future, infectious wastes may be regulated as hazardous wastes because many state and local governments have already developed special regulations governing hospital wastes. To meet these future regulations, an incinerator will need a secondary combustion chamber that can provide up to two-seconds retention time when running at full capacity and is capable of operating at a temperature of 1,800–2,200°F.

5.4.5 ECONOMICS

Regional incinerators, because of increased capacity in serving several facilities, can reduce the capital costs per ton of waste and have the potential for a quicker payback (see Figures 5.8 and 5.9).

The per ton operating costs can also be reduced because fewer operators are required for a regional facility than would be required for a number of smaller incinerators located at individual hospitals. Also, a regional facility offers a viable waste disposal option for many clinics, medical laboratories, and out-patient treatment facilities that individually could not afford an incinerator but do generate a significant volume of infectious and chemical wastes.

Because of the stringent particulate emission regulations, infectious waste incinerators will require air pollution control systems including acid gas control because of the chlorinated plastics in the waste. These systems will add to the costs.

KEY:
Capital Costs
  a With Heat Recovery &
     Ash Removal
  b With Heat Recovery
  d No Heat Recovery or
     Ash Removal Costs

Annual Operating Costs
  c With No Heat Recovery
  e With Heat Recovery

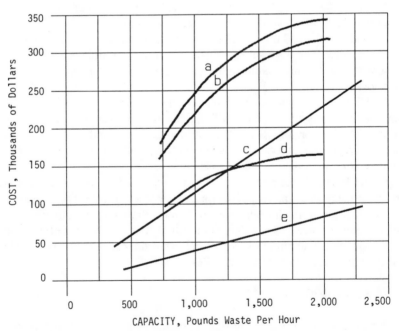

Figure 5.8 Capital and operating costs of a controlled-air incineration system in 1984 dollars. (Data courtesy of the Simonds Manufacturing Corporation.)

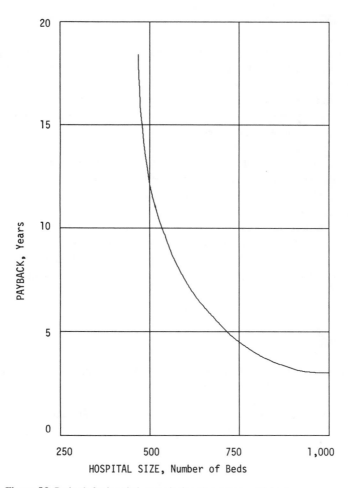

Figure 5.9 Payback for hospital waste incinerator system with heat recovery.

If the incinerator is to be permitted as a hazardous waste incinerator, a sophisticated particulate/acid gas removal system will be required. Traditionally, a Venturi and absorber system has been used, but today, a dry scrubber/baghouse system could also be considered.

A regional hospital incinerator could be an attractive alternative compared to local infectious waste disposal by offering several advantages over multiple individual units, including cost, efficiency of operation, and better environmental control. A regional unit also has the potential for energy recovery that may be more attractive because of the increased size and more consistently uniform mass flow rate.

5.5 SUMMARY

When possible, recovered energy can make the incineration system an economic asset that also treats waste material. This is especially true for facilities where large quantities of infectious wastes with high heat content are available on a consistent basis. Heat recovery, on the other hand, could create more problems than it is worth for smaller facilities even though it is often a bonus with large facilities.

Incineration system emissions must be measured and operating parameters monitored. The actual emission testing is probably best accomplished by contracting a testing firm. However, the facility should be capable of supervising the test and coordinating operations to achieve the most accurate test conditions.

Incineration is only one option for treating infectious waste. If understood, it can be a good, safe, low-cost option. The owner/operator, with the help of consultant engineers, can achieve successful treatment of infectious wastes and retain good community and environmental relationships.

REFERENCES

1 Radian Corporation. *Hospital Combustion Study—Data Gathering Phase*. EPA No. 68-02-4330 (October 1987).
2 Wood, R. W., R. E. Bastian, J. M. Osborne, A. Sigg and J. D. Wilson. "The Right Regime," *Mechanical Engineering*, 11(9):78–81 (September 1989).

Troubleshooting Guide for Baghouse Air Pollution Control Systems

T HIS chart lists the most common problems that may be found in a baghouse air pollution control system and offers general solutions to the problems. There are a number of instances in which the solution is to consult the manufacturer. This may not be necessary in plants that have sufficient engineering know-how available.

Where the information applies to a specific type of baghouse, the following codes are used:

RP . . . . Reverse Pulse
PP . . . . Plenum Pulse
S . . . . Shaker
RF . . . . Reverse Flow

Symptom	Cause	Remedy
High Baghouse Pressure Drop	Baghouse undersized	Consult Manufacturer. Install double bags. Add more compartments or modules.
	Bag cleaning mechanism not adjusted properly	Increase cleaning frequency. Clean for a longer duration. Clean more vigorously. (Must check with manufacturer before implementing.)
	Compressed air pressure too low (RP, PP)	Increase pressure. Decrease duration and/or frequency. Check dryer and clean if necessary. Check for obstruction in piping.
	Repressuring pressure too low (RF)	Speed up repressuring fan. Check for leaks. Check for damper valve seals.

Symptom	Cause	Remedy
High Baghouse Pressure Drop	Shaking not strong	Speed up shaker speed. (Check with manufacturer—could be effect of leaking primary damper.)
	Isolation damper valves not closing (S, RF, PP)	Check linkage. Check seals. Check air supply pneumatic operators.
	Isolation damper valves not opening (S, RF, PP)	Check linkage. Check air supply on pneumatic operators.
	Bag tension too loose (S)	Tighten bags.
	Pulsing valve failure (RP)	Check diaphragm. Check pilot valves.
	Air volume greater than design	Damper system to design point. Install fan amperage controls.
	Cleaning timer failure	Check to sse if timer is indexing to all contacts. Check output on all terminals.
	Not capable of removing dust (condensation on bags)	Send sample of dust to manufacturer. Send bag to lab for analysis of blinding. Dry clean or replace bags. Reduce air flow.
	Excessive reentrainment of dust	Continuously empty hopper. Clean rows of bags randomly instead of sequentially (PP, RP).
	Incorrect pressure reading	Clean out pressure taps. Check hoses for leaks. Check for proper fluid in manometer. Check diaphragm in gauge.
Low Fan Motor Amperage/Low Air Volume	High baghouse pressure	See above.
	Fan and motor sheaves reverse	Check drawings and reverse sheaves.
	Ducts plugged with dust	Clean out ducts and check duct velocities.

Symptom	Cause	Remedy
	Fan damper closed	Open damper and lock in position.
	System static pressure too high; duct velocity too high; duct design not proper	Measure static on both sides of fan and review with design.
	Fan not operating per design	Check fan inlet configuration and be sure even air flow exists.
	Belts slipping	Check tension and adjust.
Dust Escaping at Source	Low air volume	See above.
	Ducts leaking	Patch leaks so air does not bypass source.
	Improper duct balancing	Adjust blast gates in branch ducts.
	Improper hood design	Close open areas around dust source. Check for cross drafts that overcome suction. Check for dust being thrown away from hood by belt, etc.
Dirty Discharge at Stack	Bags leaking	Replace bags. Tie off bags and replace at later date. Isolate leaking compartment if allowable without upsetting system.
	Bag clamps not sealing	Check and tighten clamps. Smooth out cloth under clamp and reclamp
	Failure of seals in joints at clean/dirty air connection	Caulk or weld seams.
	Insufficient filter cake	Allow more dust to build up on bags by cleaning less frequently. Use a precoating of dust on bags (S, RF).
	Bags too porous	Send bag in for permeability test and review with manufacturer.
Excessive Fan Wear	Fan handling too much dust	See listings above for "Dirty Discharge at Stack".

Symptom	Cause	Remedy
Excessive Fan Wear	Improper fan	Check with fan manufacturer to see if fan is correct for particular application.
Excessive Fan	Buildup of dust on blades	Clean off and check to see if fan is handling too much dust (see listings above for "Dirty Discharge at Stack"). Do not allow any water in fan. (Check cap, look for condensation, etc.)
	Wrong fan wheel for application	Check with manufacturer.
	Sheaves not balanced	Have sheaves dynamically balanced.
High Compressed Air Consumption (RP, PP)	Cleaning cycle too frequent	Reduce cleaning cycle if possible.
	Pulse too long	Reduce duration. (After initial shock, all other compressed air is wasted.)
	Pressure too high	Reduce supply pressure if possible.
	Damper valves not sealing (PP)	Check linkage. Check seals.
	Diaphragm valve failure	Check diaphragms and springs. Check pilot valve.
Reduced Compressed Air Pressure (RP, PP)	Compressed air consumption too high	See listings above for "High Compressed Air Consumption".
	Restrictions in piping Dryer plugged	Check piping. Replace dessicant or bypass dryer if allowed.
	Supply line too small	Consult the design.
	Compressor worn	Replace rings.
Premature Bag Failure—Decomposition	Bag material improper for chemical composition of gas or dust	Analyze gas and dust and check with manufacturer. Treat gases with a neutralizer before they enter the baghouse.
	Operating below acid dew point	Increase gas temperature. Bypass and start-up.

Symptom	Cause	Remedy
Moisture in Baghouse	Insufficient preheating	Run systems with hot air only before starting process gas flow.
	System not purged after shutdown	Keep fan running for 5–10 min after process is shut down.
	Wall temperature below dew point	Raise gas temperature. Insulate the unit. Lower dew point by keeping moisture out of the system.
	Cold spots through insulation	Eliminate direct metal line through insulation.
	Compressed air introducing water (RF, PP)	Check automoatic drains. Install an aftercooler. Install a dryer.
	Representing air causing condensation (RF, PP)	Preheat repressuring air. Use process gas as the source of repressuring air.
High Screw Conveyor Wear	Screw conveyor undersized	Measure hourly collection of dust and consult manufacturer.
	Conveyor speed too high	Slow down conveyor speed.
High Airlock Wear	Airlock undersized	Measure hourly collection of dust and consult manufacturer.
	Thermal expansion	Consult manufacturer to see if design allows for thermal expansion.
	Speed too high	Slow down speed.
Material Bridging in Hopper	Moisture in baghouse	See above. Add hopper heaters.
	Dust being stored in hopper	Remove dust continuously.
	Hopper slope insufficient	Rework or replace hoppers.
	Conveyor opening too small	Use a wide, flared through.
Frequent Screw Conveyor/Airlock Failure	Equipment undersized	Consult manufacturer.
	Screw conveyor misaligned	Align conveyor.
	Overloading components	Check sizing to see that each component is capable of handling a 100% delivery from the previous item.

Symptom	Cause	Remedy
High Pneumatic Conveyor Wear	Pneumatic blower too fast	Slow down blower.
	Piping undersized	Review design and slow blower or increase pipe size.
	Elbows too short radius	Replace with long-radius elbows.
Pneumatic Conveyor Pipes Plugging	Overloading pneumatic conveyor	Review design.
	Slug loading of dust	Meter dust in gradually.
	Moisture in dust	See listings under above section "Moisture in Baghouse".
Fan Motor Overloading	Air volume too high	See below listing for "Air Volume Too High".
	Motor not sized for cold start	Damperfan at start-up. Reduce fan speed. Provide heat faster. Replace motor.
Air Volume Too High	Ducts leaking	Patch leaks.
	Insufficient static pressure	Close damper valve. Slow down fan.
Reduced Compressed Air Consumption (RP, RR)	Pulsing valves not working	Check diaphragms. Check springs. Check pilot valves.
	Timer failed	Check terminal outputs.
High Bag Failure—Wearing Out	Baffle plate worn out	Replace baffle plate.
	Too much dust	Install primary collector.
	Cleaning cycle too frequent	Slow down cleaning cycle.
	Inlet air not properly baffled from bags	Consult manufactuer.
	Shaking too violent (S)	Slow down shaking mechanism. (Consult manufacturer.)
	Repressuring pressure too high (RF)	Reduce pressure.
	Pulsing pressure too high (RP, PP)	Reduce pressure.
	Cages have barbs (RP, PP)	Remove and smooth out barbs.
High Bag Failure—Burning	Stratification of hot and cold gases	Force turbulence in duct with baffles.

Symptom	Cause	Remedy
	Sparks entering baghouse	Install spark arrestor.
	Thermocouple failed	Replace and determine cause of failure.
	Failure of cooling device	Review design and work with manufacturer.
Bearing Failure	Overheating (temperature, measured by a bearing-temperature detector, is in excess of 90°C or, when measured by a thermometer at a point on the bearing housing nearest the bearing, is in excess of 60°C)	Replace/fill oil reservoir. Clean oil rings. Resize/replace bearings. Redesign shaft arrangement.
	Worn out or dirty oil, insufficient oil; oil rings jammed; excessive end thrust or misalignment; excessive loading conditions	
Bearing Housing Oil Leak	Vent in housing plugged sealing compound omitted from housing surfaces; incorrect grade of oil	Replace/fill oil reservoir. Reseal housing.
Electrical Insulation Failure	Moisture, dirty metal particles, or other contaminants on the insulated windings; power sources; excessive temperatures; mechanical damage; voltage surges; excessive vibration with resultant mechanical damage	Heat environment. Filter air. Use regulated power supply. Redesign mechanical components.
Motor Failure; Excessive Vibration; Noise	Misalignment; uneven air gap alignment; settling of foundation; parts rubbing the rotating element; sprung shafting	Tighten anchors. Replace foundation. Balance. Check shaft. Align.
Will not accelerate	Wrong connections; open circuits; starting voltage; excessive line drop; excessive load; mechanical obstruction	Check wires. Replace starter. Resize motor. Redesign unit.

Incineration System Field Inspection Report Cross/Tessitore & Associates, P.A. Environmental Engineers

CHECKLIST FOR INFECTIOUS WASTE INCINERATOR FACILITY

Administrative Information

Facility Name:_____ Address:_____

Telephone: (_____)_____ _____, _____ Zip:_____

Permit Information

Air Permit: ☐ Yes   ☐ No   Expiration Date _____

Special Provisions (i.e., monitoring, temperatures, etc.) _____

_____

_____

RCRA-B Permit: ☐ Yes   ☐ No   Expiration Date _____

Special Provisions (i.e., monitoring, temperatures, etc.)_____

_____

_____

Inspection/Enforcement Activity

Last Regulatory Inspection: Date: _____ Inspector_____

Agency: _____

Violations Noted? ☐ Yes ☐ No What? _____

_____

Violations Corrected? ☐ Yes ☐ No What? _____

_____

Violations Not Corrected: _____

_____

Time Table to Correct Violations: _____

_____

Performance Conditions

Parameter	Permitted Condition	Observed Value
Burnout:	_____	_____
Opacity:	_____	_____
Temperatures		
Primary:	_____	_____
Secondary:	_____	_____
Loading Rate:	_____	_____
Combustion Efficiency:	_____	_____
		Last Stack Test (Date: _____)
Emissions		
Particulate:	_____	_____
HCl:	_____	_____
Other:	_____	_____
	_____	_____

_____   _____

Company Performing Tests: _____

Incinerator System Information

Incinerator

Manufacturer: _____ Type: _____

Model Number: _____ Rated Capacity: _____

Date Installed: _____

Primary Chamber (Design):   Temp._____   Res. Time_____

Secondary Chamber (Design):   Temp._____   Res. Time_____

Air Pollution Control System

Does incinerator system have bypass?   ☐ Yes   ☐ No

If yes, how often is it open? _____ per month,

and for how long? _____ min. at a time.

Manufacturer: _____   Type: _____

Model Number: _____   Capacity (acfm): _____

Residue Management

Incinerator

−sprayed?   ☐ Yes   ☐ No

−quenched?   ☐ Yes   ☐ No

−EP Toxic?   ☐ Yes   ☐No

If yes, why? _____

_____

_____

Air Pollution Control System

−EP Toxic?   ☐ Yes   ☐No

−Are bottom/top ash mixed?   ☐ Yes   ☐ No

−If yes, is an ash EP Toxic?   ☐ Yes   ☐ No

If yes, why? _____

_____

Disposal of Residue

Name of Hauler: _____ DOT I.D. #: _____

Landfill Receiving Waste

Name of Landfill: _____

Type of Landfill: ☐ Mono fill   ☐ Reg. SLF   ☐ HW LF

Permit No.:_____

Expiration Date of Permit:_____

Container Used for Disposal

Type: ☐ Drums   ☐ Totes   ☐ Other: _____

Size: (yds.) _____

Are there fugitive emissions?   ☐ Yes   ☐ No

Are fluids leaking from containers?   ☐ Yes   ☐ No

Waste Handling/Storage

Waste Delivered in: ☐ Bags   ☐ Boxes   ☐ Other: _____

Is cold storage provided for delivered waste?   ☐ Yes   ☐ No

If yes, how long is the waste stored? _____

How is waste fed to the incinerator?

☐   Cart dumper into hopper with ram feeder

☐   Manually into unit (no feeder)

☐   Manually into hopper with ram feeder

List any operating problems with system.

_____

_____

_____

List any maintenance problems with system.

_____

_____

_____

Housekeeping and Environmental Information

Drainage Problems?   ☐ Yes   ☐ No

If yes, specify source of odors. _____

Noise Present?   ☐ Yes   ☐ No   If yes, specify source of noise? _____

_____

Is waste handled effectively?   ☐ Yes   ☐ No   If no, why? _____

_____

Operator Training

Is operator trained?   ☐ Yes   ☐ No

If yes, then how trained?   ☐ OJT   ☐ Schools

Does the operator have creditation?   ☐ Diploma   ☐ Certifications

  If yes, from whom?_____ Date: _____

  Explain amount and quality of training. _____

_____

Insurance Coverage

Type Coverage   *Amount Per Incident*

Employer's Liability   ☐ Yes   ☐ No   If Yes, Amount: _____

Comprehensive General   ☐ Yes   ☐ No   If Yes, Amount: _____
Liability

Comprehensive   ☐ Yes   ☐ No   If Yes, Amount: _____
Automobile Liability

Environmental Impact   ☐ Yes   ☐ No   If Yes, Amount: _____
Liability

Citizen Complaints

Have complaints been received?   ☐ Yes   ☐ No

If yes, list nature of complaints and number. _____

_____

Index